Dedicated To
Trevor Brian Matthews
5th March 1954 – 28th July 2001

Thank you for being my Dad

When I'm feeling weak
And my pain walks down a one way street
I look above
And I know I'll always be blessed with love

Contents

1. Introduction
2. The Why
3. Fundamentals
4. Mindset
5. Movement
6. Macros
7. Madness
8. Marriage
9. Money
10. Moving Mountains – The Everest Obsession
11. Putting It All Together
12. Small Stuff, Big Results
13. The Three Phases
14. What Is It Really Like To Lose 100lbs?

1. Introduction

'Look, if you had one shot, one opportunity, to seize everything you ever wanted, in one moment. Would you capture it, or just let it slip?'

Eminem said that way back in 2002 and to be honest back then life was so good. It was so easy to stay in shape there were no worries, family to take care of businesses to run but now. Wow, life has changed a hell of a lot. Some days the joints feel like they want to stay in bed other days the brain wants to stay in bed with the joints taking the dogs for a walk. That dreaded sound.

'eeeh eeeeh eeeh eeeh'

The slap of the sleep button.

'eeeh eeeh eeeh eeeh'

It's time to get up but you really want to chuck the duvet back over your head and drift back into that dream you were having running down the wing on cup final day at Wembley, 100% fitness in the prime of your life without the spare tyre fit for the latest hybrid SUV stuck round your waist.
Jump up, first part is the worst, that pissing mirror you have to walk past that hides nothing. Summer is the worst time as you

don't even wear your pj's it is straight up boxers (with the hems rolled over thanks to the muffin top sitting above them) this is real life, you've let it slip prioritising the things that most men pride themselves on.

Family.
Business.
Friends.
Life.

Well you aren't alone:

OVER 65% OF MALES IN THE UK ARE OBESE
(www.noo.org.uk 2014)

That is a shocking fact and honestly when I was searching knowing it would be high I never even thought it would be that high.

Even more shocking.

YOU COULD FILL THE ENTIRE POPULATION OF THE UK WITH THE OBESE MALES IN AMERICA – AND STILL HAVE OVER 10MILLION PEOPLE SPARE.

That is why I wrote this book.

I'm giving you the simplest plan to work out how to make the change. One day at a time. Upgrade your body taking one step after the other after all...

'A journey of a thousand miles starts with just one step' – Lao Tzu

There are so many books out there that go into ridiculous depth, giving you every technical term under the sun you need countless hours on Wikipedia in order to understand half the content. It is time that there was something that you can not just reference, not just read and leave but also have with you ready to upgrade your body, your life and also give you that easiest way to implement everything we go through whilst understanding WHY you have been doing the things you've been doing getting where you have gotten to and make those feelings simply just memories.

Now as mentioned this book is going to give you a full plan by the end of it you will have the answers to:

• Why you do the things you do and how to over come the blockages
• Why you self sabotage your progress and how it is just an excuse
• Why your family are your biggest excuse
• How to fit everything in even if you work 25 hours 8 days a week

- The perfect day based around all the fundamentals of The One Day Body Upgrade

This will be given in simple easy to understand terminology so if you are one of these people that wants to know the entire backlog of science from Einstein to Hawkings from Edison to Newton and so on. You won't get the entire functions from the body in depth that you need a degree to even be able to pronounce the literature, that is what I have spent years researching, implementing and finding out working with hundreds of clients all around the world to bring you the basics of what works because after all, life should be simple so you can live it to the fullest right?
It won't give you a massive in depth plan specifically tailored just for you as that is what I work in depth with together with my clients on a daily basis but it will allow you to form your own day. It will give you the answer to totally upgrade yourself with the only side effects being that you thrive day in day out with your family, friends, and business.

Is this really for you? Let me ask you this. Did any of that ring true at the start? Are you that person? Do you find yourself tired in the morning but wide-awake at night? Do you have time to give all the attention to your children that they deserve? Do you have the time to please your partner?

Can you even still 'please' your partner…?

Have you tried all the diets around, fads, exercise plans, have you been that 300 rep Spartan or that circuit training dude that got booted out of boot camp because you struggled to even tie your own trainers in the car park before the session started. The guy sweating because they are out of shape in the staff meeting, who can't even get up the stairs at work in the morning without getting out of breath. Do you really want to take the lift? Are you the guy who gets that new membership contract at the gym January 1st but next time you go to the gym you turn away because you can't get the parking space that is closest to the door?

This is for you if you are one of the business men, entrepreneurs who want the best out of not just your business but your lives, wanting to thrive but right now you are part of #TeamNoSleep and working 25 hours a day 8 days a week and can't take that family holiday you need so much, hell you can't even have your anniversary off. You've hit the limit to what you can achieve, you're successful in your business but in doing so your health has dropped you live on a diet of nootropics along with a side of extra strong coffee to make sure your productivity is up, is that really what you want to be living like for the rest of your working career, No? Then this is for you.

Imagine this:

You're 35 years old and what should be the 'prime' of your life, but you aren't, you aren't even reaching 50% of your potential, you've put on around 10kg these past 12 months.

You do nothing.

You hide away.

You continue getting heavier.

Your fitness keeps dropping.

Eventually comes a heart attack.

You survive, just.

What then?

What do you need in order to change?

Imagine looking back, you're 50 years old and right now are 35 you didn't change ANYTHING. What would your 50-year-old self tell you?

Think about that for a minute.

What if you only had to focus on one day at a time?

It will hurt to truly admit it to yourself that you need to change.

But honestly, I cannot force you. You can keep lying, you can keep hiding it but it's your life. If you are truly happy with your health 100%, if you truly have got everything you can want out of your business, if you are happy with not being able to see your children grow old because you are slacking on your health right now, that's totally cool.

I understand.

Put this book down IMMEDIATELY.

Still with me?

So why now and why not 5 years ago?

Well here's something I learnt a long while back and is the secret of changing for the better.

PAIN

You have to be in enough pain or even this in the words of Tony Robbins –
"Change happens when the pain of staying the same is greater than the pain of change"

So you have to really be in pain, and by that I don't be you've broken a leg been shot in the knee and had to sit through each episode of Made In Chelsea back to back, no. I mean you have to be really pissed off by the position you have got yourself into, yes YOU have gotten YOURSELF into, nobody else has done it. This is where we are going to delve into in the coming chapters. And the great thing is that we are going to also show you how to build your perfect day and overcome those blockages. We will go through the fundamentals – The 3 M's – Mindset, Movement and Macros in order to show you how to build your perfect day, the small things which make the biggest impact to your life, and in turn not just yours but your family too.

Have you every heard the analogy 'fix your gas mask first'? When you are in an airplane and they go through the safety procedures, life jacket, wings, exits here, here, and here then the gas mask dropping down, you need to fix that gas mask before you help your family if not YOU won't be able to breath and YOU won't be able to survive so YOU won't be able to help anyone around you unless YOU have that focus on YOU first off. So, in short, we are going to be showing you how to fix your gas mask first.

Why me?

I'm that dude that you may have seen on social media that has been in shape and has it easy right? Wrong, I have been ridiculously out of shape I am talking to the point I had to drop over 80lbs, to the point I would need my inhaler not just going up the stairs but by the time I got to my car at the end of the driveway, actually I lie and I admit it, that's an understatement, it wasn't even at the end of the driveway it was parked right by the door. Tying my shoes was an issue, just bending down my gut would get in the way, it was not pleasant, but what really rubbed it in and caused me to shove a hypothetical firework up my arse was when I had a reality check.

Reality check time:

I was due for a meeting, the lifts were broken and I had to go up 4 flights of stairs. I drove in that morning it wasn't hot it was like November and I parked as close as possible. Got my morning coffee, two sugars chocolate dust on top and walked to the meeting, I had to stop halfway for a breather then I got to the meeting it was embarrassing and I kind of hate it still to this day, there was a ridiculous sweat patch like my shirt had melted to me, it was bloody freezing outside like to the point people had coats and scarfs on to walk in from their cars! This wasn't nice. To top it off it was a meeting with the big guys for a promotion, yes I once had that 9-5 corporate job you guys live on a daily basis and wanted to progress too. Safe to say my first impression sucked arse as much as sucking arse can actually get, this was one of the most uncomfortable and horrible moments in my life and I had to change.

That night I went in and looked seriously on myself, I invested in help, my own personal trainer but not only that I read every single book I could get my hands on. Loosing weight was hard, gym work was hard, getting my life in check was hard.

NO – these were all predisposed beliefs I had told myself this was all bullshit. Why? Because being embarrassed to the point you want to walk out of the room and quit your job was even harder, to the point everyone was speaking about you and no one wanted to sit next to you due to risking getting sweat flicked onto them as it dripped down your back and onto a sweaty arse print on the plastic chair, this was reality, this was my pain, this what when it became a lot hard than the pain of change and I had to do something about it.

I haven't looked back since and dropped the weight I needed, as a result I was able to inspire others to do the same, build my business up with what had become my passion and no longer was sport just a game that was played on the PlayStation in the evenings it was something I was able to get my hand in, I have since then worked with athletes all around the world bringing what I have taken on board to my day to day clients, to my online clients and transferred these learning's to information which now helps people just like yourself, you don't have to be a bloody marathon runner, a triathlete, a power lifter, boxer, bodybuilder you just have to be willing to put in the effort because you are seriously pissed off with where you are right now. This has been why my one day body upgrade methods have been so successful in helping business men just like yourself in following suit changing their lives to the point where they are proud and not just proud but healthy.

My only question to you is this:

Are you honestly happy with no just how you look but how you feel right now?

Let's get things moving.

2. The Why

'When I'm feeling weak, And my pain walks down a one way street. I look above, And I know I'll always be blessed with love'
– Robbie Williams

Why?

We all have a 'why'. That small thing we don't realise is there until we dive deep into our subconscious and realise it's actually a massive thing, driving us in the direction we are passionate about in life. Do you know your 'why'?

This may be the most important chapter of this book but it's nestled right at the end, why? Well, I am going to tell you my 'why' and I didn't want any judgement going through – I know, I have said for you not to worry about judgement but I kind of wanted you to believe I was just in this because I had gone fat to thin and now just love working with busy guys because you know, money.

That is not my why.

Let me ask you this.

When was the last time you spoke to your dad?

Mine was when I was 15, actually it was 21st July 2001 to be exact, when I physically spoke to him on the phone, I text him on 23rd July 2001 if you want an exact contact date.

I never knew a life where my mum and dad were together, they split when I was about 5 years old, I remember my dad dropping me off and I would sprint from the back door to the window on the stair banging on the window crying my eyes out waving goodbye to him as he drove off in his then blue Ford Capri (he loved that car!) he was going off to work a little further away than the city we lived in, about 30 minutes drive as a caravan salesman. I remember that we would have to wait and maybe would see him some weekends and on a Sunday night he would give us £3 in 10 pence pieces to play on the amusement park on the seafront, then I would go to school and see both parents picking children up, my friends would be there with their parents on their birthday every year as I grew up, I only wanted that – my dad to be with me on my birthday as I opened presents, my dad to be with me on Christmas morning when I opened presents, surely it wasn't much to ask? But my dad was out there in the stressful life he was living not bowing down to targets but rather making sure he hit them month after month in order to provide for his children, that made him proud.

After a few years he went from salesman to sales manager to the point he actually took over a park near Colchester 'Weeley

Bridge', this was about 90 minutes away at least (but we got to stop off at Burger King so that was cool!) now we would only see Dad during school holidays, maybe a week at a time, it was getting further and further apart as he worked harder and harder to provider for his family, the stress was hitting him hard, migraines were happening regularly but it didn't stop him, he turned the park around and got moved to one on Mersea Island even closer to Colchester, I know I took so much from my dad and his determination to succeed, it was unrivalled.

Coopers Beach on Mersea Island was the last park Dad worked in, he went on a training course in July 2001 in Grantham near Nottingham, it was here where he was messing around playing volleyball after the day's antics had been completed and got a paralysing migraine and he was taken into hospital on the Wednesday, something we were apparently being protecting from knowing by our aunt and uncles, it was how the family was bought up I suppose but then on Thursday 26th July 2001 my dad suffered a stroke where over half of his brain was essentially killed, oxygen was starved for 13 minutes – to this day I want to blame someone but everyone was just doing their best, doing their job, trying to help my dad but they couldn't .

We got there on Friday 27th July about 11am with my family gathered in a waiting room there were no words to say what needed to be said, we all knew what was going to happen, it was just a matter of time. I remember even to this day what I was wearing, black shell suit kind of material trousers, a wu-tang top with the W in red with a red NY Yankees cap on, I remember where everyone was sitting, I remember the smell, the sound of the machines and the look on the nurses faces every time they came in to see how we were doing, no words were being exchanged it was just what I thought was 'a blur' but in reality it was 100% focus, this 15 year old boy was losing his hero, the guy he adored, his father and I remember the feeling when we knew it was all over. I was invited to say my goodbyes, walking into that ward seeing my hero, pipes in him, not moving, being kept alive my the machines buzzing, beeping, motionless, time was standing still, this was it. I slowly walked up to the side of the bed, the far side, all this time I was wishing inside of my head 'someone wake me up now, wake me up'. I held my dad's hand, slowly bent towards his ear and whispered.

'You're my hero dad, thank you, I will make you proud'
July 28th we had to make the decision for the life support machine to be turned off, 21:50 my dad, Trevor Brian Matthews passed away.

Stress killed my dad.

Stress killed my hero.

Because of stress my dad never saw his children finish school.

Because of stress my dad never saw my sister and I drive our first cars.
Because of stress I never got to take my dad out for a pint at 18.
My dad never got to see his children graduate from university.
My dad never got to walk his daughter down the aisle.
My dad never got to share the top table at my wedding.
And, because of stress my dad never got to hold my neice, Eden Sofia Grubb in his arms when she was born on 5th November 2016.

So when people ask my why?

Why do you work with business guys, busy, stressed out entrepreneurs, people who have so much on their plate they need a second side dish and an extra doggie bag just to cope.

Why?

Because if I can stop ONE child going through what I had to go through at 15 years old then I am complete.

I won't lie, it has brought me to tears typing this but as you will know from the previous chapters, emotions make us strong, hiding them is what stops us from moving forward.

Thank you for reading.

3. Fundamentals

"If you spend too much time thinking about a thing, you'll never get it done" – *Bruce Lee*

So you're still with me right? Good.

Let's go through the fundamentals, get you really ready for what is going to be happening as you go through this blueprint, show you where the changes will be implemented and the real progression of fulfilling your potential.

We will briefly touch on the 5 M's here and start to really find your reason why but not just that also the reason that the media has been failing you by putting out bullshit article after bullshit article just to sell stories and scare people into different tactics.
After all, life if for living right, not for reading the damn newspaper day in day out or scrolling through Facebook finding the latest viral blog post that everyone is cringing over.

Mindset –

Where else would we start?

Let's try something here, I want you to think back, like way back, to when you were a baby.

Remember it? No?

Because you were thinking and living in the moment, no memories to stop you from doing things, nothing that was scaring you, just you, an innocent young soul in a body real to learn so many different beliefs that other people had been taught years ago that moulded them into who they were which were ingrained into their parents and mentors years before. Nice to be told what to think, what to say, what to do and how to live isn't it.
Well that is essentially what we learn growing up and now I want to look to see why this is stopping you from reacting your full potential.

The mind is a wonderful thing, it can scare you, it can make you happy, it can make you sad. But it is just that, a mind, inside a head, inside a brain that inevitably you should be able to reason with and not control as such but have some sort of influence over.

What is a tree? It is a big piece of wood made up of a trunk with branches coming out, leaves and potentially fruit, maybe some bloom from those branches but we are going to look a little deeper and see the beauty in learning to control the roots day in day out.

But what actually is it? Is it a tree, or is it the opinion of someone who chose to call it a 'tree' many generations ago and has done all the thinking for us? Sounds a bit far fetched hippy crap but stick with me on this one we will go a little deeper into the mind when we reach the mindset chapter.
The mind is a wonderful thing, that is, when we are able to use it for positive and progression. When you understand what you are actually doing you can become aware when you are in a mode of 'self sabotage' or 'self love' (don't think what most people think there, please)
I'm not here to give you all the answers but I am going to give you the ability to find them for yourself , no one can give you the answers, in fact, you already have all the answers deep down as to why you aren't in the shape you want to be or at the level you want to be.

We are going through the fundamentals right now so I will hold back on depth and detail but when you master the mind you will easily get your head around the main three parts I work with when I delve into client reasons for wanting to get where they want to get:

- Motivation
- Determination
- Realisation

Those are three powerful words. Without the first two you won't ever get the last one.

If you aren't motivated you won't have the drive and determination to see it through. If you don't believe you can get the realisation you won't have the motivation and determination to see if through, we could go on.

We are bought up on beliefs, again this will be delved into further but here's an example that I have personally had to deal with.

My Mum doesn't believe I can earn good money helping people transform their lives, she says she does and she supports me (which I have no problem in believing at all) but she was bought up in a world where you were cautious, my Nan was very hard up in her words she was bought up 'in a slum-ouse with 12 brothers and sisters' (she had the strongest Norfolk accent I have ever heard) she had to share a bath and her parents got the water last, 12 people to share a toilet, there wasn't much wealth in the family so it is understandable to have some caution. However when I decided to jump ship and stick the middle finger up at the corporate way of living where I had to book my holiday 2 years in advance and work a shift pattern that meant I missed the most important days of the families lives, my Mum was dubious – that life was safe – the life I had been close to redundancy twice because of budget cuts and off shoring NOT down to my own performance – that life was safe – I had a contract but that life I reiterate WAS SAFE, that was the belief here. You are with a company your future isn't in your own hands but you are safe. I really feel this is how 90% of the population think down to my own interactions and experience. Going self employed and living the life I dreamt I could do and envisaged every time I see my Mum now she is worried 'are you doing ok' in reality I am earning a lot more than I did at this corporate company working less and even when I am 'working' it feels like fun. But that is the belief – you HAVE to live how others live because it is safe.

I guarantee when we dig deep down that you are not where you want to be because you have told yourself you don't deserve to be there, and you tell yourself it is ok, you are happy.

But, in reality, you aren't happy.

Movement (and Macros)–

This sounds obvious but to burn those wonderful things we call calories we have to do this special thing called moving. Moving burns energy, but what do we mean when we are talking about movement?

Movement isn't just what we do when we are exercising it is built into our day left, right and centre. It is a matter of developing habits and again, being present and aware (awareness is going to come up a hell of a lot in all of the chapters we go through here) of the decisions we are making. Choices are everywhere, just so happens we get a little lazy in those choices.

I am not just talking about walking to work instead of driving. Let's go a little deeper here of the different choices you can make related to walking instead of driving to work:

- Walk instead of drive
- Park further away
- Stairs not lifts
- Use the bin furthest away
- Use the printer furthest away

Simple things but just being aware throughout will add to this movement. Again we will go into depth of how to utilise the movement potential of your body.

As with the mind we have three movement parameters to cover – Strength, Speed, Stamina and every movement we go through in life will involve a certain aspect of each one just at differing levels throughout. Every goal you have whether it is to run a 5k park run to running the London marathon, squatting your own bodyweight to competing in a power lifting competition, beating that bloody old person who makes swimming look so damn easy and effortless at 6:30am every morning or swimming the first discipline in an Ironman triathlon. You will require a certain amount of strength, speed and stamina and to be honest it won't just be in movement we require some of these, you still will need a certain level of strength and stamina in order to hit your goals elsewhere including in the kitchen, let's not forget the strength when out with friends for the Friday drink.

But how should we move?

Everyone is different as we know and everyone will want a different outcome, I will go into an analogy when we get to the macros but let's put it in your mind already.

Not everyone wants to build a massive castle with thick walls, some people will want a lean functional sky scraper, some will want a small facility that is hassle free and doesn't require much maintenance, we will go through your goals and how to go about them, the first steps and consistency.

How do you get those houses built?

The Macros

I've heard this in different terms over the past few years and macros in short make up most of our food choices.

Now whether you have heard it made up in a term such as If It Fits Your Macros or just as a pointer in the different types of food that are going to make up your nutrition. Macros make up a vital part of your body upgrade and are the final one of the 'Three M's'

Carbohydrates, proteins and fats are the three macronutrients and eating too much of one and not enough of the others won't get you where you want to be, eating too many of all of them won't get you where you want to be. We will workout based on your goals and movement amounts exactly where we need your focus to be and the balance we need to have between each macronutrient.

As important as macros are there isn't much to say in regards to the fundamentals as we will cover so much when it comes to the actual chapter further on in the book, that's is where we really get into the meat and two veg of it (literally).

What if you don't want to do it?

Well, simply, don't again I invite you to put this book down if you feel you are exactly where you want to be, stay there and don't progress. That's cool. But if you are ready to do the most important thing you ever can do then I am excited to be a part of that. Are you ready for the biggest step of your life?

TIME TO TAKE RESPONSIBILITY.

We can blame our ancestors, we can blame our parents, the ex girlfriend, children, friends, media. But with all due respect, you are where you are right now because of no one else but yourself, that is the harsh reality of life unfortunately. No one held a gun to your head and said to sit down with that takeaway and eat it whilst drinking a 4 pack of beers on the side. No one done that but you. It is simply a choice you make to have junk food or have good food that will help you on your way. It is simply your choice to skip the gym because you are tired due to eating crap, sleeping late and having that long day at work eating chocolate raisins on the desk all day long. It is simply up to yourself to take responsibility and I am not going to try to polish a turd in this book I am going to put it just as it is, taking all the science out of it and say it in plain English how to take responsibility and get to where you want to be, well, where you SAY you want to be anyway.

Media Myths

Unfortunately some of the things we have been bred into thinking aren't always down to our pure ignorance they are down to the crap we are fed left, right and centre in the media. Now, some people may have different views on this but I am going to be straight up, I have nothing to hide here in telling you what I believe.

Carbs are bad –

No, that is very incorrect. Over the years we have been made to think that carbohydrates are the devil out of the three food groups, I won't go into the depths that some books will but basically carbohydrates are used within our bodies in order to give us energy, they provide practically instant energy for us to use, unfortunately some people eat too many carbs, carbs are nice and very VERY easy to eat so it is understandable. When carbs get processed sometimes the body won't like them as much but again as long as you are getting about 80-85% of your carbohydrates from good single ingredient whole foods (we will go into food quality and types during the macros section) then you won't go far wrong, providing you aren't allergic or intolerant to any specific things you are eating.

Sugar is the devil –

Again like carbs we are taught that sugar is bad, in essence no, no it isn't the trouble we get is that some foods are again very processed as mentioned previously. These processed foods won't do the body as good as getting good whole foods in there and in moderation if you do want a few sweets it is totally ok, if sweets are a bit of a trigger then I would steer clear for a bit.

Cholesterol is bad –

We have two types of cholesterol in our body – LDL (Low density lipoprotein) and HDL (High density lipoproteins), LDL being what is known as 'bad' and HDL being known as 'good'.

First off when a doctor does a test unless requests in detail it is usually just a total cholesterol marker meaning the total of both of the two put together, now this would be good although let me ask you this.

If a football game had 6 goals is it a close match? Maybe, but it could be 3-3 or 5-1 one is close one is a white wash.

This is the problem with having a total cholesterol test, you may have loads of HDL and little LDL, I would always request a full cholesterol test if you consult your GP.

Also 90% of the time dietary cholesterol (that age old thing that eating too many eggs will be bad for you – yes, that is another myth) will not raise your LDL levels, that will be down to lifestyle, genetics, loads of alcohol, smoking and junk food. Let's just get that clear now.

Fad Diets –

I'm pretty passionate on this subject so I will just keep it simple that way it doesn't have to last about 50 pages long – Diets based on shakes only as meal replacements won't work

long term, I am talking those diets that Jenny down the road sells to you who didn't know about them last weekend and is now an expert because she is part of a pyramid scheme and get's paid so has put money in front of the livelihood of her friends and family in order to destroy their health with low quality, low nutrient shit that quite frankly has not even got a 'plus' to any 'life' at all I don't care who that body is by. Nutrition and health should be a lifestyle, it should be something you don't have to have as a fad but things you can live with day in day out.
9 times out of 10 these fad diets will be dropping weight ridiculously quick, most of that weight will be water weight meaning you feel horrendous with bags under the eyes and look like you're about to audition for the next Resident Evil film. What happens when they start eating 'normal' again? They put on more weight than they had when they started, potentially actually doing long term damage in the process – I think I made my point there.

Cleanses and Detoxing –

Unless you are munching on loads of factory waste products, have a side of AA batteries and a cocktail of petrol, oil and gas mixed together then your kidneys and liver will easily be able to detoxify your body again without having to go see Jenny and her latest pyramid scheme which will are pack with so many 'superfoods' turn you into a Superman within 7 days. (Let's not start on 'superfoods')

Unless you have predisposed medical conditions then this will always happen alongside a couple of other things – a good balanced diet, doing a little bit of exercise regularly and drinking that magic liquid we all source from turning a tap – water.
I think this goes with the fad diet part – there are no quick fixes.

As we continue I will go through some more media myths throughout the book, give you the truth on going down the 'free from' just to drain your bank account.

Money –

Yeah, you got the money thing sorted right?

Surprisingly we all have money problems, I have said it multiple times recently to people, that guy sitting outside of the city hall in his sleeping bag selling The Big Issue – he has money problems right? Well, let me tell you this, Bill Gates, Richard Branson even Mark Zuckerberg they all have money problems, welcome to the real world EVERYONE has money problems we just need to find out what is holding us back from getting more money and honestly, 9 times out of 10 it is NOT the business that is the reason for holding you back with your bank account, this book will give you the first steps towards driving forwards with your money in order to push and create complete balance all around in your life.

Madness –

Are you mad? No I don't mean like mad as in have you turned into Heath Ledger Joker mad 'Why So Serious?', I mean are you having fun, yes, fun…madness.
Madness is about fun right, madness is putting that extra little piece into your life that gives you excitement, that piece in your life that gives you pleasure and gives an overall balance and Revitalization throughout.

Marriage –

But Why? Why now? Why me?
Everyone needs a reason if now there is no drive or motivation to make that reason a realisation. (See what I did there?)

We need to look deep down and dig, remember in the intro about the mirror and walking past seeing those muffin tops jumping out laughing at you like something off of Sesame Street? Did that hit you where it hurts?

Marriage isn't just about two people joining together at a ceremony which leaves them next to being bankrupt (why the hell does everything cost 5 times as much when you mention 'wedding'?!) it is about relationships, relationships with yourself and the reflection in the mirror, relationships with your friends, relationships with your family and relationships with your better half, we will dive into it in a lot more detail here and you can see what we really mean by this, is it really where you want it to be right now?

Listen to this for an example and see what relationships you can see are in this story about a client.

I am going to tell you about a client I had and I know it sounds harsh but I am glad we went into the office and had a chat where I made him cry.
This guy was very overweight, worked hard don't get me wrong but was over weight, he was mid 30s, since he turned 30 he had put on nearly 100lbs, he was already over weight but now he was 320+ lbs. We chatted as to why he wanted to lose weight and the obvious health came up but he knew that health was an issue and he was weak, couldn't do one push up, he was addicted to a lift of fast food and Chinese takeaways, the addiction which he had to feed. He was knackered in the morning having sugary energy drinks just to get through and it was not a nice life he was leading.
He had just got married and his Son had just been born too. This was the kick he needed. We said how he hadn't got where he wanted to be and let it slide when he was 30, this is 5 years later and he had put on nearly 100lbs in that time, another 5 years if nothing changes the chances are that he will

put on another 100lbs too, we discussed what it will feel like to get to see his Son walking to school for the first time, stepping onto the football pitch for the first time, graduate from university, get married and even become a Dad himself to which he replied that it would be an amazing feeling he can not imagine the joy – then we mentioned that in 5 years time with another 100lbs added to the already ridiculous stress the body is under the chances of him even seeing his Son go to his first day at school were slim.
He broke down.

This was the main reason why he needed to change, and from that day forth he wanted to change but it took a lot of digging in order to get him there.

I want you to think deeply, what are the reasons you want to change? We will go through these a bit more in the mindset section but find out now and be honest with yourself.

Are you single? Are you attractive to the opposite sex?
Are you married? Can you still please your other half?
Are you that guy dripping in sweat at the business meeting you own, needing to give that presentation for YOUR company and garner the respect of others but you like a wet sponge to begin with?

These examples do sound pretty extreme but us as blokes seem to pride ourselves on things like this, if it hurts it is probably something pretty close to home.

I know this from first hand experience because I was that guy who took too much interest in his job and the opposite sex would just laugh me away to the point I had to make that change, and did.

Now this change isn't something that will happen overnight but the secret is simple and will be given to you in this book. The title gives it away 'The One Day Body Upgrade' this isn't something that you get done overnight, you don't wake up a different person like Tom Hanks in big because you've put a dime in the Zoltar Speaks machine. It is simply breaking your goals down into single days which are so easy to follow it will be harder to get it wrong than get it correct.

So one day at a time right? After all, you only ever have ONE DAY. Stop all that 'Someday I am going to be fit' Someday is the equivalent to dreaming, you're not sleeping you are awake, in the present moment and ready to LIVE. And add to that, what if you did only have ONE DAY to live? Wouldn't it be better to live it to the maximum rather than hit a brick wall because you are running on empty at 3pm?

We have been through a good amount here covering the fundamentals of the process and touching on some hard to take points. We have covered 'The 5 M's – Mindset, Movement, Money, Madness and Marriage' and shown you what you will be able to create when you have finished this book.

The basics have been touched on, whilst these are the fundamentals they are also the foundation to success. We now have an idea of what your 'why' is and we will now continue in getting a route in order to deliver on the upgrade that will fulfil that 'why'.

One word I have used throughout my life and continue to use is 'honesty' something I pride myself on, everything in this book is true, if I tell you I done something, it happened, it is the only way to show you how you will need to dig and get the truth out of your own mind in order to really upgrade your life, feel great and thrive.

4. Mindset

'Life has three rules: Paradox, Humor, and Change.

- Paradox: Life is a mystery; don't waste your time trying to figure it out.

- Humor: Keep a sense of humor, especially about yourself. It is a strength beyond all measure

- Change: Know that nothing ever stays the same.' *- Dan Millman – The Peaceful Warrior*

Wow, Mindset.

I bet you've heard so many times and may have even taken on board a hell of a lot but 'mindset' is the first of 'The 4 M's' and I personally believe the most important as if this isn't correct then the other 2 at just set up to fail, I would almost certainly put money on it actually.
In this chapter I believe that you may actually finish it with a completely different outlook on life as a whole, I know, powerful words and what the fuck is Ollie talking about right now but let me explain.
We are going to go through some BIG things, focus, motivation, beliefs and why they are stopping you being everything you want, why your drive sucks and how to reverse

this, how to develop powerful habits, find a moment of realisation when you are so aware that you can tell when you are just feeding your mind bullshit excuses and honestly when I went through this the first time I had to take a walk with myself and just be one, since then my life has literally change 100%, but EVERYTHING was already there I just had to reveal it and believe and finally we go into the biggest thing that changed my life 'Motivation vs Inspiration: Goal setting 101' it should have it's own chapter but it's my book so I will just make this the longest chapter in the book due to it's importance and then touch on mindset again when we show you how to move a mountain all by yourself later on.

So let's get into the nitty gritty right now.

Focus:

What is your WHY? Why do you need focus? What is focus?

If you aren't focused then how can you progress?

Here's the deal, the road we want to travel has a start and a finish right? We are so focused on that finish we lose focus on the journey, the most exciting piece. And here's a secret, that road will NEVER be straight, it may lead down the wrong way one time or another, you may have to make a decision as someone has done some road works and popped a cross roads in the mix but that is the best thing about the journey and focus, focus is what we need to make sure that journey leads us closer and closer to our goal.

What is your goal then? Is it a business goal? Is it health? Is it family? Your goals may develop and change as you change and your journey progresses too but imagine having the single goal of finding this present moment, NOTHING else matters, right here, right now, this is all we actually have, if you can get to focus on this present moment that is an amazing feeling, that is power. Now NOBODY can add anything to this moment, NOBODY can take anything away from this moment. Focus on one thing and I am so grateful that right now that one thing you choose to put your focus in is the text in this book, for that I am thankful.

Let's look at where this focus adds up, I am going to use the Tour De France as an example.
Multiple stages over multiple weeks with the best cyclists in the world doing crazy things over ridiculous altitudes and climbs to be the leader wearing the yellow jersey at the end when the tour stops off in Paris.
This is focus in short term over three weeks but imagine how it will be if you take this focus and put it to the way you live your life.
We have different stages over this three weeks, someone wants to win he needs to focus on each of these stages, now he may not be a specialist in this particular stage, he may need to be a sprinter, a climbing expert that is great in the

mountains he needs to be overall the best rider with the most consistent focus throughout these three weeks of the tour. Now these guys have a big overall goal and need to remain focused on the overall goal as the times are added up throughout but breaking this focus down into daily stages ONE DAY at a time allows the bigger goal, the bigger focus to take care of itself.

That is what we want to get to with this book. I will walk you through everything you need we all have overall long term goals and need to be focused on those but breaking that focus down into each part of the journey, each day allows this puzzle to become so much easier to complete.

Motivation:

What is it? Honestly, so many people get motivation by so many different things, when I was 20 I was motivated by a different thing than when I was 30, in truth right now still different things motivate me and bringing my own focus into the picture allows me to keep this motivation up each day, let's not beat around the bush here EVERYONE will have days they feel like total SHIT, when things don't workout the way they want it to work out, that is called being human, if people tell you otherwise they are just bullshitting you I guarantee. But the good thing is when you know what your mind is doing, where your motivation lies and where your focus is, you can EASILY become aware (as we will go into later in this chapter) and snap out of it getting back on track and staying 100% motivated about 99% of the time.

Even nutrition is seemingly hard to get motivated on, we see quick fix diets because people don't want to be drawn into the long term now imagine this, you have your nutrition everyday sorted, sorted specifically for each day at a time this is so much easier to take than knowing you have to eat boring stuff (which it won't be even for this one day) every month for 6 months just to get rid of those muffin tops. Training for example, you don't need to do 60 sessions (5 times a week for 12 weeks) you just have to have the motivation for one session which is based around your schedule, you're business I get that, your schedule only allows 30 minutes to do some movement 'thing' for 4 days a week, that's cool, we are only going to be doing it once a day, there is only one day we need to focus on, and as we build this knowledge up (which is already inside your head) you will learn that one day is all you need to be focused for and nothing else matters it's like groundhog day but only a bloody amazing feeling living the perfect day every day.

Beliefs:

Wow, this is one where I literally took so much on board I didn't know where I was or what I believed. You don't have to go that deep but let me put things into perspective.

We go to school – we are taught every day 5 days a week then 2 days where no doubt we will be doing homework from the age of 4-5 years old until 16 moving on to college and university levels some people will be learning from other people's OPINIONS for even the first 24-25 years of their lives, then they go to work to do tasks which have been created by another person's opinions and beliefs for the rest of their lives until they retire around 65 years old.

We are taught opinion, from people who have been taught someone else's opinions who got it from the opinion of the generation before and I could continue but you see where I am going with this right?

Why are you scared? I have been asked this so many times and I had a discussion with someone yesterday. This guy had a massive role in the army previously and had to jump out of planes at like 20,000ft in the air he mentioned he was scared the first time it happened. But what if you had no doubt the parachute would open, you would land in the correct place you didn't get fired upon by the enemy got picked up and returned home safely. You had NO idea these things could happen only you had been fed since you were a toddler that jumping out of a plane is fine along with your parachute opens all the time with no mechanical issues EVER, I mean, you've never actually had a mechanical right? Fear gone because you have followed a different set of beliefs.

Let's look at another example of a belief with fear as an underlying theme. You walk out the door, lock it, open the gate, get in your car, reverse off your driveway and go off to work, normal day. You aren't scared at all here right? But what if you had been taught to believe that just walking out of the door you are potentially going to get massive hail rocks drop at you from the sky trip down the driveway and your car roll on top of you because the handbrake is crap meaning you suffer career ending injuries paralysing you for the rest of your life (extreme yes I know), in all honesty this is actually just as possible as a mechanical happening with the parachute opening but you aren't taught to believe this could happen but it could, you just don't believe it could happen. That is a belief based around fear.

A belief I have dealt with time after time again is that one my Mum engrained into me as a youngster – I need to be in a 'safe' job, you know, one with a contract and a boss type thing to tell you what to do. I used to be in a 'safe' job in the corporate world. My day would be as follows:

Wake
Go to work
Follow rules and orders along with systems someone else BELIEVED would work best
Go home
Sleep
Repeat

But this was 'safe' because it was the belief in society that you had a 'cap' on your earnings based around someone else's opinion and couldn't get any further.

Now this safe job may I add I lost two management positions not down to performance but because someone else had their beliefs and believed they needed to cut the budgets drastically and also send a whole department off shore. See what living by someone else's beliefs and rules leads to most of the time?

Now back to what happens now years down the line after I have carved my life seemingly out of my own beliefs. When I see my Mum nearly every time she asks with a certain degree of worry if the business is doing good, in reality it's bloody thriving and I love every day helping people it feels so much better than being the top selling person in the insurance industry, but I have managed to live my own beliefs and we will develop your own set of beliefs carving out your 'perfect day' by the end of the book too.

It is awareness, which will let us see these beliefs, and you will actually be aware as to which are your own and which are other people's beliefs, the greatest thing of knowing these beliefs is that you will stop them becoming 'self-limiting' and be able to really thrive off of your daily routine loving every second.

I'm going to tell you of another belief I heard when listening to an audio book before but honestly this has stuck and the title hasn't:

A guy was having sausages on his 'sausage night' of the week, his wife used to chop the sausages in half all the time, he thought nothing of it as this was normal then one day he asked her
'Why do you chop the sausages in half' bemused the wife looked at her husband and replied
'Because my mother used to do it'
'Why does your mother do it?'
'I'm not sure you will have to call her'
The guy called his mother in law up and asked the question again
'Why do you chop the sausages in half'
'Well, it is because my mother never used to be able to afford a large frying pan and my father liked sausages all cooked at once so to fit them in she had to chop them in half, I just continued as it was normal'

Makes you think how many other things we do mindlessly because it is 'normal'.

Determination and drive is a big thing (I suppose it is all BIG so to speak!) and pretty similar when it comes to motivation linking in closely with realisation too. But it is so much easier to have the determination to finish one day than it is to finish one month if you look at a marathon as 26.2 miles it's hard but if you look at it at 1 mile 26 and a bit times the mind can comprehend it a hell of a lot easier. That's the same as life itself, well I find it a lot easier to focus that way, the same with working out, even with determination at it's fullest I still focus on client's and their ability to 'trick' the mind it isn't 12 reps it is 1 rep 12 times, counting down from 1-6 and then 6-1 it seems such a shorter set and gets completed near enough 100% of the time.

Determination is defined in the dictionary as 'the process of establishing something exactly by calculation or research.' Now if you calculate what you want to do with your life it is one of the hardest things to muster up and stick to, for starters how long are you going to be alive? 50 more years? 30? 20? 10? Even longer? How long until you 'retire' if you even want to be able to retire? 20? 30? 40 years? Now if we can only 'calculate' enough determination to be able to live ONE DAY at a time, this is where life really gets an upgrade.

Think of it like this.

Motivation is what gets you going.
Determination is what keeps you going.
Realisation is what you get when you are well on your way each and every day at a time.

We will get to realisation in a minute but first off I want to let you into the biggest development that won't just help you with your health but also your life, your business, your family and overall your entire body upgrade.

Habit.

Habit development is crucial here and so many people base their entire 'programs' on 21 days, why? Because that is how long it takes to do something in order for it to become a habit. I believe this is incorrect. It doesn't have to be 21 days, there are 24 hours in a day, why can't you develop habits in 21 hours? Imagine developing a new positive habit every day of your life, a step ONE DAY at a time in the direction you want to be going. This is simple.
Screw 21 days, that is too long, it tells my mind I have time to waste, time to wait and time to burn. No, I don't and I know this for a fact. People fail with their habits because they take far too long to develop because we are taught again because of someone's belief that it takes 21 days in order to create a habit.

The habit is already there, the behaviours are already there, the only time you have to develop your habit is 'now' this present moment. It is why I am a massive believer in habits being a present. Habits cannot be developed in the past and the damn sure can't be developed in the future they can ONLY be developed NOW, this present day is where you will develop your habits, so in that sense it is NEVER possible to develop your habit in 21 days.

But what is a habit?

Again we can look at the dictionary definition and we find it is a 'noun' 'a settled or regular tendency or practice, especially one that is hard to give up'

Imagine creating your ideal life through your own body upgrade and daily habits, after all how great with it be that it is actually going to be HARD TO GIVE UP?
Once we get our brain trained into believing and knowing it has something to do, each day, it locks in on that habit, we are going to create your perfect day but in all honesty we should call it 'your perfect habit'.

Realisation

Imagine realising every day you wake up that the day ahead of you is pushing you forward both mentally and physically in not just your life but your business too? You have learnt how to believe, set goals, achieve and now upgrading your body NOTHING will be able to stop you, I guarantee.
One person described realisation to me as the conversion of assets, goods or services into cash or receivables through sale – I think they got that from the dictionary too but imagine that. If you know why and how you are motivated, have the

determination to do this then you will get realisation in a hell of a lot more money but not just the you will receive much more ability to use the world's biggest commodity which we cannot buy more of – time.

Realisation is exactly what it says but just being present allows you to feel and take it in over and over, this is the beauty of it all. The experience is realisation. And when it all clicks, which it will as it has done for clients all around the world already, you will notice that motivation, determination and realisation just blend into one, a kind of 'zen'.

Before I get too hippy chick lovey dovey shit on you.

Why can't you do it?

Go on, ask yourself that.

Why?

Why can't you get in shape?
Why can't your business thrive?
Why can't you have so much time with your family you have to take them to Disneyland multiple times a year and take selfies with Mickey?

Let it settle for a minute.

Ok, do you know why?

Really?

Because you are full of excuses and mental blocks which actually deep down are guilt for other things.

That sounds so harsh but I know it is true and mean it in the nicest possible way, after all I said I wouldn't sugar coat anything.
When we tie our excuses down we can almost certainly link them in to when someone else fed us a belief.

You can't earn money doing the job you love – feed that back to my Mum's belief as mentioned earlier.
You can't lose weight – the person who told you that can't lose weight very well, doesn't have the ability to focus (show him this book please!)

Some of them we tell ourselves because of a lie.

I HAD to have a Chinese – no you didn't you had forgotten to shop, weren't prepared and couldn't be arsed to get decent food out and plan, not an issue having a Chinese meal at all as long as you put in the work all those other days beforehand and know it will potentially have a 'step backward' effect, but if you're upgrading your body each day then that's cool because you will be more than two steps ahead beforehand.

I HAD to have that drink – no you didn't, your friends peer pressured you into thinking you can't have fun without some alcohol, this isn't your belief it is theirs, they THINK you will be boring without alcohol, in truth you won't, they won't remember and you will have more money and actually enjoy that fry up the next day rather than puking it up immediately afterwards when you wake at 2pm which will then mean you're hung-over and struggle to get up creating that 'Monday morning feeling'

These are just two excuses or blocks people believe in because of not wanting to be man enough to stand up themselves to even people the call 'mates' or stand up to their own laziness. I'm not being harsh it's just true, I know this because I was that person and it took a massive amount of realisation to get there.

The truth is we all will have times we eventually lack a little motivation and determination but if we know you have had the realisation at one point then it is so much easier to get back on providing you are also upgrading your life ONE DAY at a time, if you know what motivation is it is easier to see when motivation is slacking, if you know what determination is it is easier to see when determination is slacking, it really is that simple. It is all a matter of 'awareness' whether you like it or not, present moment living allows you to be in a constant state of awareness, no I don't mean as if you've popped 50 stimulants and chucked loads of LSD into the mix on a night out (don't do that, I never have I was trying to be funny and majorly OTT there but I can imagine you will be pretty aware of being 100% unaware!)

As I will go through this a few times and link it to each chapter, awareness is a big thing to be able to control, if you are aware when you are doing things you can change, if you are aware when you aren't doing things, you can also change. You can create a positive awareness and change for the present moment lifestyle to really allow you the ability to automatically 'upgrade'.
I want you to try this little exercise and be 100% honest with yourself. It may hurt I am not even going to lie on this one – to be honest I can't remember the last time I lied apart from when the wife asks 'are you listening?'

Write down 10 excuses you have had – let's not use the word excuse here actually, write down 10 reasons you aren't where you want to be, these may not be down to your own fault – notice the important word there being 'may'. I won't be able to see them but I will be more than happy to check in an email if you pop them over to Ollie@revitalizationblueprint.com we can go over them further if you like.

Let's go over this a little more with depth now and one way I know works with my clients day in day out, it's kind of a 'Goal Setting 101' a tried and tested method which actually has had multiple people breakdown into tears when they imagine not hitting their goals, it's powerful for more than just your health, trust me.

We've looked at why you want to do things right? Well, let's change the wording there, when we tell the brain different things our subconscious will latch on with certain wording even with a weight loss goal for example 'I want to be 90kg' it's very specific and get's the brain thinking 'oh it's so specific I can't stay at this for very long' or even 'ok I am 90kg now I am stuck' and you don't get to improve from there – If you set yourself a goal range the brain kind of get's tricked 'I'm not going to get stuck at a weight, watch me move forwards and get within this window, less stress for me for certain!' Visualisation techniques here are being used for a weight but the most powerful time I use them with clients is asking why and what if and if not they actually do certain things, we always ask ourselves this:

'What happens if it doesn't work?'

Have you ever asked yourself this?

'What happens if it DOES work?'

So you have your specific goal, let's use one of them for example weight loss.

What happens if you hit your goal?

You will feel great, more confidence, sex drive up, be earning more, be more focused, health markers have improved and you will be feeling so much more comfortable in your clothing.

OK, so flip it.

What happens if you DON'T hit your goal in the time given?

You will feel deflated, still no confidence, still uncomfortable in clothes, still not able to please your wife in the bedroom department, you will still be having to dive into the disabled toilet at the top of the stairs to pinch the hand dryer to get rid of the sweat patches off your shirt from walking 50m from the car to the door (in the middle of winter WITH NO RAIN FALLING DOWN) oh and your child will still be saying 'I love Daddy's rolls on his belly' alongside you will definitely still not able to run around for 30 minutes with your children without making an excuse to sit down or 'I'll go in goal' to get your heart rate back down to 'not quite about to have a heart attack' levels.

What's the WORST that could happen if you DO hit your goal?

This is big, hard to answer unless you look deeper into it, so for weight loss it will be something along the lines of – I won't be able to fit in the clothes now (too big), may have to worry about birth control methods ;-), your children will be so proud of you saying 'look at my Daddy's abs' not flabs, you will get looked at by those 'chicks' whilst driving with the hood down in the centre of town on the summer's day and you may even get mistaken for being Christian Grey or Daniel Craig when you're ordering your Martini, shaken, not stirred. We really are pulling things out of not a lot here too with what is the worst that can happen so, let's flip it.

What's the WORST that could happen if you DON'T hit your goal?

Your wife leaves you, you have a heart attack, you have a stroke, your children grow up wanting nothing to do with you, your confidence drops lower, you lose your financial strength, the business falls apart, you put on MORE weight from stressing about it, your sex drive gets even lower and even, death, yep, I did say it and the truth hurts.

So there you have one massive eye opener, I remembered some big things just going through it with you and that is what I love about this sort of stuff, you already have everything you need to be so successful, you already are that successful upgraded businessman but you just need to reveal it first off to yourself then to the rest of the world. You are aware of what motivation is, determination and realisation you know how to be aware of blockages, examples of excuses, you even know why most of the things you believe now are not your fault they may not even be your parent's fault, of your grandparents but generations before them that put certain thoughts into their mind, it really is time to start thinking for yourself and as the guy did in the example JUMP THE FUCK OUT OF THAT PLANE!

5. Movement

'Take action! An inch of movement will bring you closer to your goals than a mile of intention.'
— *Steve Maraboli,*

I believe that sums it up, we have nailed the mindset, we know no what your goal is, there is only one way to get there, movement.

So many people have the intent to move, the intent to hit their goals but action speaks a hell of a lot louder than words.

So what do I mean by movement? I mean LIVE, BREATH, THRIVE, PROSPER. Some of the things in life that really upgrade you all achieved through movement. Movement is exercise but we don't have to see it at exercise in itself, but more habits that seamlessly flow in and out of your daily routine. By the end of this chapter you will see how you can change little EASY habits that will make so much difference in your life and getting you closer to those goals.

What do you want to get from movement?

That's a big question, we could answer in typical 'male testosterone' fuelled statements and say 'I want to bench 100' or we could answer in real person terms 'I want to be able to thrive in my business and live to see my daughter graduate'

I prefer the second one personally as I have had so many seemingly healthy guys that I know (not clients!) have to miss important family events because their health suffered and that's not even starting with they inability to fulfil their business potential too. Something I want to change wherever possible. Something I hope this book allows to have a positive impact not just on your life but the family that you support each and every day.

So let's start off with something basic. You more than likely have an iPhone or an android, now these things will easily track your steps, if you want to get even more specific you can get apple watches, fitbits and many other fitness trackers which you wear on your wrist. Keep the phone in your pocket and see on an app like My Fitness Pal how many steps you walk each day roughly.

There is a magic number but as we know, everyone is different so I would start to consistently aim for 10000 steps per day just for health, then, aim to find things you can change in order to increase this output. Even 100 steps a day before you know it you're on 11k steps, then 12k and so on. You won't even notice it I guarantee.

How do you increase these steps? Simple ideas such as walking to work if possible rather than driving, or riding instead of walking, ok you may not have loads of time so we have other ideas. Most of the high flyers at the office have a special spot near the door, screw taking your spot, take the one furthest away you will get a good few hundred steps extra easily. Also take the stairs instead of the lift even if it is just one floor, well worth it. If there are toilets you use further away than the normal ones, go walk to those during the day. If you make a drink and have the option of a kitchen a couple hundred steps further away again go for that kitchen, do you see where I am coming from here?

Goes the same when out shopping, pick the supermarket car park space furthest from the door and trolley park. Pick the cinema parking space on top of the multi storey instead of the one by the door, and use the stairs.

See what I am getting at here?

Get some goals, develop habits and the steps soon add up.

You are a bodybuilder

'Every sport is bodybuilding in it's very essence. You are building your body for a specific purpose, for a specific sport. We can all learn from the details as long as we know the end goal'

This is a true statement in all aspects of life and for every single sport on the planet, why? Because you are building your body for a purpose, for a goal. If you are a businessman you want to build your body for the goal of thriving and building your business to the top end of the totem pole, you want to be at number 1 in the standings, you want to get on the Forbes list and you can build your body to cope with the stress you have to deal with on a day to day basis, building this body will also have to able to be constructed in short spaces of time, maybe hotel workouts as you are on the road, maybe short 15 minute full body sessions first thing in the morning each day, we want to build that body with as little negative impact to your business and lifestyle and the biggest maximum impact you can get.

STRENGTH>SPEED>STAMINA – TECHNIQUE (triangle)

We have three focuses with movement.

Strength, speed and stamina 'The Three S's' and each of these needs a certain amount of technique which is specific to really thrive.

Now this isn't a big textbook where I will go through lifting technique or even how to program your training for strength if you are a powerlifter or stamina if you are a long distance runner. I have worked with 100s of athletes 1-1 and I do program so get in touch if you would like this (Ollie@revitalizationblueprint.com) but right now we are focusing on keeping it simple, there is no way you will find any of this complicated if you focus on one day at a time.

Strength –

What is strength?

Some people would define strength as the amount of weight you can move over a certain distance from A to B – 'How much you bench bro?'
Some people would define strength as a mental aspect
Some people may define strength as something different entirely but for now let's look at a day to day life of you as the successful business guy you are, oh and that family guy, remember that time you got tired putting your child over your head, that time they were like.
'Daddy, do it again, again, again'

The shoulders were burning and now your child has grown a little you struggle to even lift them up. Ok, not many guys will be lifting their 21 year old Son up, although if you have a daughter you may want to have the strength to throw their first boyfriend halfway down the street!

This is strength in it's basic form, day to day strength –

- Lifting your briefcase when it's full
- Taking the shopping out of the boot
- Moving furniture
- Picking up the Rottweiler when it's no longer that tiny puppy
- Lifting up your children
- Even opening the door can be a struggle for some people.

This is what we need to do, the basics, not lift 100kg over and over again, and that is what I focus on with clients.

Try this for each day so simple but it will allow us to see where you are at.

Day 1 Press ups until you can't do any more, then straight away into bodyweight squats all the way down for 3 minutes.

Day 2 Press ups with 5 less than before but repeat this 5 times with the same number of squats immediately after each set (so if you got 25 press ups you will then do 5 sets of 20 press ups then 20 squats after each set)

Day 3-9 repeat day 2

Day 10 repeat day 1 and see the improvements

I guarantee you improve. So simple yet so effective.

Speed

This is the second 'S' and just as important as strength.

What is speed? Most people will define it as the time it takes to get from A to B.

I suppose in the correct term it is this and will stay true to this any way we may look at it. But let's put it into real terms where we need speed.

- You're late for your meeting, you need to get there quick but not be a stinking sweaty mess by the time you are there.
- You are pretty close to missing the train and have to run to the next platform
- Your car ticket is running out and the traffic warden is right there about to write a ticket .
- Your children have done a runner at the beach and you have to catch them up.
- You are playing football with the kids and you have to tear down the wing.

These are just some real true to life examples of speed.

Speed will come with building up your strength and I do have tips on how to interlink this will building your stamina too which will definitely not break the bank or destroy your daily time keeping.

Here's a little session to do where you will just need some trainers.

Lamppost sprints

You can get the little one to time this if you wish too.

On the pavement find one lamppost and you will be able to see not the next one but the one afterwards SPRINT to it and get the child to time you.
Wait 20 seconds then sprint back, you must always beat the previous time.
Wait 20 seconds and repeat again 20 times.

This will help you develop your speed, we will look to increase this with a client after a couple weeks and have them doing this 3 times a week at first, when increasing I would go to 3 lampposts rather than 2.

Stamina – The Final S

Just as important as the other two so it isn't a case of 'best until last' scenario here, each links into the other. If you haven't got stamina you won't then recover quickly with your strength or speed and vice versa.

What is stamina?

It depends who you ask but most women will tell you that you need more of it as a man. That's a big kick in the balls trust me!

Stamina if we looked at it in a real life situation like the other two will be things like:

- Simply walking and not having your shins pump up and calves start hurting, let alone your lower back giving in.
- Simply standing up without having to lean over or grab the nearest chair.
- Stamina is found in the bedroom (needed anyway!)
- Stamina could be how long you are able to concentrate in the latest meeting .
- It is how long you are able to play with your children, you don't want to get knackered before they do, imagine how they would feel.
- It is even being able to walk the dog at the weekends.

We could continue but I think you get the picture, stamina isn't just about running the London Marathon it's about taking the kids to school, doing real life things I mean, it's cool to have a formula 1 car but you still need something road legal to go to the shops in right?

Stamina is something we build up daily and as you increase your steps you will increase your stamina, as you increase your strength your stamina will increase alongside if you increase your speed your stamina will also increase too.

With all of the 'Three S's' we have something that crosses over which really separates the good from the great, which will really set you aside from the rest when upgrading your body, it's kind of the development of a specific habit which makes you increase your skills in each S, technique.

Technique is developed by your body learning motor patterns, I coach technique in both the physical and mental form. Technique isn't just something we look at physically but in developing physical technique your mind will become primed in order to develop it's own mental technique and this will crossover to the habits you develop and do without even realising in the kitchen too.

Remember when we were talking mind-set how we went over awareness? Well, awareness is a pretty big thing we need to look at here with movement too. If you aren't aware of what you're doing then how can you change it?

We have the step counting as one of the first steps of becoming aware; one thing that helps so much with awareness, which my clients have told me, is that they invested in my help with 1-1 coaching to become accountable. Being accountable will work wonders for your awareness trust me, let me put this into a form you will DEFINITELY be able to understand. Remember when you were like 12 years old and you used to leave your television on, radio, light and the tap running and your Mum would shout 'wait until you have to pay the bills' well, that day came right? Not a care in the world about how much electricity or water you were wasting until you got an estimated reading then you was like 'shit I need to give the actual readings and stop wasting energy'

That's accountability and awareness, you are aware that the outcome is wasting a lot of money because you have to pay for it. Find something that allows you that amount of awareness and you are on to a winner.
Easy Lifestyle Swaps

Just implementing a few little swaps in to you day to day life can increase your activity a hell of a lot immediately. Simple things such as:

- Take the stairs over the lift – even if you're only going up and down a couple flights it can add a few hundred steps on to your daily total which will then add thousands over the year, they all add up.

- Park further from the door – When we get higher up in companies and even in our own companies we reward ourselves with closer parking spaces, is this really a reward, damaging our health? If you park further away even if it is only 100 metres or maybe on the floor higher in the car park you will rack up so many more steps per day and it will only take a few more seconds to get to the office door.
- Don't order online – This is convenience at it's best, we have been spoilt but years ago there was nothing like 'online shopping' there wasn't 'one click checkout' shops didn't deliver your weekly shopping to your door in a convenient 1 hour slot, we have become lazy and it suits us because we have let it, we always used to have the time but now we say we don't have the time anymore. Actually doing your shopping, pushing the trolley around the store, going to buy your clothes rather than mail order all of these things don't exactly cost any more, in fact they may cost less with no postage fees to pay but they all allow you to increase your day to day step total, this is what we want.
- Adjustable desk – this is a good one but not something many people do, first thing is getting an adjustable desk, not too expensive but it will allow you to stand whilst working for a couple hours a day all the time burning more calories and getting healthier throughout.
- Do away with your chair – a little like the adjustable desk but actually having some time off of your chair

and on an exercise ball will allow you to activate vital core muscles and not only help your posture but burn calories throughout without even knowing.
- Walk to work- so many people, and I have been guilty of this a lot in the past I will admit this now, will walk to work when in reality they live only around 25-30 minutes walk to the office. Ok in winter time it may be dangerous if it is icy, it may be raining heavy but in summertime the weather will be pretty much guaranteed to be spot on for you to be able to walk to work so there really isn't an excuse here.

So there we have it, the simplest things can get you the furthest in health and developed your One Day Body Upgrade. Focus on moving as much as possible, implement these tips into your daily routine and you will be well on your way. There are so many fitness trackers around but on mobile phones and watches so there really is no excuse not to be able to track how much you are moving. A good target is at least 10,000 steps on top of any gym session you may be doing each day it sounds a lot but it really isn't.

We have the basics to follow and know that movement isn't just getting from a to be but rather The Three S' we have Speed, Strength and Stamina and depending on your goals the amount of each of these required will differ from person to person but in an ideal world we will all have a good amount of all three of these.

Get on top of each one at a time and you are more than well on your way.

6. Macros

'The proportion of ingredients is important, but the final result is also a matter of how you put them together. Equilibrium is key.' – Alain Ducasse

Macros.

Otherwise known as 'macronutrients' basically these are the main bulk of what we eat made up of carbohydrates, proteins and fats. (Alcohol technically is a macronutrient but the body can't really do too much with it!) We need these in full and I will briefly go through this chapter in order to let you know why you need each one and what some good sources of each one would be. I won't be going into detail of what your calories will be and depth of the actual structure of your diet as that is something I go into depth with in the plans I create for my clients (we can talk further at Ollie@revitalizationblueprint.com). What I want to make sure you leave this chapter with is a basic guideline of what is and what isn't going to be optimal for your nutrition and totally implementing your One Day Body Upgrade.

Protein/Carb/Fats/Calories Infographic here

The simple rule – when picking your food sources the quality of food will make so much more difference than just the individual macros in the food you have chosen. Picking good 'single-ingredient' foods will mean they aren't processed and have all the quality and goodness kept in them that will make sure your body is able to thrive each and every day in your body upgrade.

It is also good to note that if your overall calories are too high it won't matter how much you follow the individual macronutrient guidelines, your body won't be in a calorie deficit so you won't lose weight.

Protein:

One of the most commonly known food groups it seems and is usually associated with muscle-bound lumps that live in the free weight area of the gym posing at the mirror all day long whilst taking a selfie for their instagram account.
Now protein is vital for everyday life, every living strand in your body is essentially protein and without this we wouldn't be able to survive very long due to our body not being able to recover and repair all the cells in our bodies.
Protein is made up of individual amino acids some of which are created in the body and some which are essential to be included in our diet, this is why it is vital to make sure you get enough dietary protein in order to meet these needs.

Now, it is common for anyone to overestimate their daily protein needs and if you overeat that is cool no need to worry too much despite what the media will have us believe as providing you have no other issues your kidneys will just help the body deal with it, you just may make a little more body 'gas' during the day, always good to clear the office lift!

Protein is commonly found in animal products, meat, fish, eggs, dairy and also in good amounts in nuts, soy, tofu all containing different amino acids some sources will include all of the aminos too. What I advise my clients is to make sure you get a good amount of varying sources throughout the day in order to make sure you get plenty of these amino acids and don't then get deficient in any throughout.

I would always recommend a client to get just under 1 gram of protein per pound of bodyweight but also aim for the target bodyweight so if you are 200lbs and you want to be 180lbs then you should set your protein around 160-180 grams per day roughly. In each gram of protein there are 4 calories so this will mean you would get 640-720 calories per day from protein here.

Carbohydrates:

I love carbs! No, seriously they are the meaning of life I swear! So many people I know have demonised carbohydrates but essentially carbs are actually the source of energy for day-to-day life and will be the centrepiece in your body upgrade.

Carbohydrates are what will go into your muscles and also take water in there, allowing the muscles to function and give you the energy not just to perform but also the allow your brain to function optimally too.

There is a myth that eating carbohydrates after 6pm will make you gain weight, this is false, overeating calories at anytime will make you gain weight. People also find they drop weight quickly when they go low carbohydrate and there is a specific reason for this – For every gram of carbohydrate in the muscle the body will also bring in 3 grams of water too that means when you take carbohydrates out of the body you will also take out 3 times the weight in water. The trouble here is that the body needs to be hydrated and by taking that water out your brain function will drastically decrease, not good for business! And once the body has got rid of the water and your performance in the workplace and even the bedroom hits rock bottom, your weight loss will halt too.

Carbohydrate sources again are widely known but just for clarification they can easily be found in foods such as potatoes, sweet potatoes, pasta, bread, rice, couscous and oats amongst a lot of others. Also we find some sources are fibrous carbohydrates, which are also essential for our body, and we will go into these a little bit in the next chapter when we cover the 'small big things'.

When structuring your diet I like to go for about 2-3g of carbohydrates per pound of target bodyweight when you are training, some athletes I will have up to 4 or 5 grams. So that means if you are around 200lbs and you want to be 180lbs you would look to get about 360 grams of carbohydrates on a training day minimum. In each gram of carbohydrates there are 4 calories just like protein so therefore you would get around 1440 calories from carbohydrates here.

Also I advise clients to get their carbohydrates in around the periods in the day that they are the most active. Whilst the body won't really just store carbohydrates as fat if it needs the calories it is always good to plan your nutrition around areas of the day when you will need higher energy.

Fats:

Fats have been demonised just as much as carbohydrates over the years, we need fats to survive, that again is a fact. Fats are great, they help with hormone production and also they are greatly required for joint health too.

We have different fats such as saturated, unsaturated and trans fats. The media has given saturated fats a very bad rep over the years and links it with high cholesterol levels however no matter what, if you are a healthy individual with no predispose health conditions then eating dietary cholesterol will not increase your blood cholesterol levels, things that would increase cholesterol are things like a sedentary lifestyle, a lot of smoking and drinking along with a diet full of junk foods so if you fit into most of those categories then you really should get started on the advice I give you in this book.

Fats will be found in abundance in items such as nuts, eggs, fatty meats, oils, butter, oily fish and things such as avocados too.

Unsaturated fats are the fats which are usually liquid at room temperature such as olive oil and unsaturated fats come in two types both polyunsaturated and monounsaturated fats. It is wise to get a good source of fats in the diet as it will help you provide the body with things called 'omegas' which are numbered 3,6,9 and are essential for overall health in the body.

When you have checked out your required protein and carbohydrate amount the way to find out how many fats you need is to find your overall calorie need, take the calories out for protein (4 calories per gram) and for carbohydrates (4 calories per gram) and then divide the remaining calories by the calories in fats per gram (9 calories). I will also make sure that this isn't less than 10% of the total calories and ideally at least 15% minimum.

Here's something that really helped me get across to some of my clients the need for having the right amount of each macronutrient in your day to day nutrition.

Think of it like this, protein are the bricks, carbohydrates are the workers and fats are the cement. If you don't have enough bricks the workers aren't able to work, if you don't have enough of a work force you won't get the bricks into position and if you don't have enough cement you can't build the solid base and get the bricks stuck together.

Now this also works with too much of something – too many bricks will mean just a mess on the front garden and turn to rubble, too many workers and they will just hang around looking ugly and out of place and too much cement will mean that it will just set again on the front garden becoming solid and hard to move.

How Do You Fit It With YOUR Lifestyle?

Now, you are a busy guy, I get that I really do but we all have the same 24 hours in the One Day of our body upgrades. We will always want to make the most of those 24 hours, after all, time is the one commodity we cannot ever buy any more of so we need to be prepared. Whether that means you prepare your food once a day or you prepare it in bulk, whether that means you get someone to prepare it for you or know where you are going to buy it each lunchtime or get it delivered to you each day, preparation is key.

When selecting your foods it is important to take into account what facilities you have at your disposal throughout the day and choose foods which will allow you to still enjoy your food along with being able to get the most out of it too. What I mean by this is if you really can't stomach cold chicken and you don't have access to a microwave then don't have cold chicken in there and put something you can stomach in there. If you know you're going to be in and out of meetings then having little snacks like nuts and protein shakes will be a lot easier to have throughout, you can always have a drink in a meeting. If you spend a lot of time on the road then finding good things at service stations will be needed, you can prepare food for 2-3 days but any more and it would potentially just go off.

Set yourself up for success this is going to be key. You don't have much time so getting your head around food preparation will help no end, you can even get companies that deliver your food to your door fresh for the week, these are great but I personally prefer clients knowing exactly what is in their food and learning how to make it themselves. Here are some great ideas as to how to maximise the use of your time when preparing food, eating out and getting through the work day.

- If you have a grill such as a Foreman grill then use tinfoil, you won't have to clean it really very often and can just through the foil away afterwards.
- On the subject of the grill if you are going to cook your chicken portion then cook multiple amounts of chicken, as many as you can fit on your grill, myself I wrap a portion in tin foil and can get 4-5 servings on one grill, meaning I have it prepared for 5 meals from one use of the grill.
- Batch cook other things in tin foil such as potatoes and sweet potatoes, again you won't need to prepare the food more than once simply chuck them in the oven for a good amount of time (usually 45 minutes to an hour) and then wait to cool and chuck in Tupperware tubs then keep them chilled in the fridge, they will last a good 3-4 days easily.
- Cook vegetables in bulk, I literally fill my steamer with vegetables enough for a good 3-4 days again, I get mine frozen but fresh works just as well, filling the layers of the steamer and putting it on until cooked through throwing the cooked veg into the Tupperware boxes again.
- If you have a portion of 75g rice uncooked then cook up 300 grams and simply spoon it into 4 different Tupperware boxes, you don't even really need to worry about weighing it just put a roughly similar amount in each box, you will be eating the same amount over the

course of the time anyway so a few grams extra or less in one meal won't break the bank.
- Plan ahead – again this goes with the preparation subject but if you are going to be travelling then get some fruit and protein shakes in, same with meetings if you are going to be in the meetings so you aren't tempted by the biscuits and sweets that inevitably get thrown in the middle of the meeting rooms just grab a serving of nuts and a protein shake, you will be instantly upgrading your body by doing so.
- When you are due to eat out, decide what you want to have beforehand and do not ever hesitate to ask to have your food served a certain way, so many people have allergies and intolerances nowadays that asking for your steak to be grilled plain is not a problem at all, asking for potatoes without any oil or butter on them will not be an issue, you are paying for the food you like so it is your choice how it is prepared.

Throughout this chapter we have gone through a lot of information around what foods are great, at the end of the book there will be a guideline layout of how to structure your day food wise so please make full use of this, ok it isn't tailored to your specific tastes and daily routine, get in contact to discuss us working together in order to get a plan specific to yourself (Ollie@revitalizationblueprint.com).

You can see from this information if you pick whole foods which really haven't been tampered with much you can't go far wrong in all honesty.

7. Madness

"See what I mean? You gotta be crazy. Ain't no time to be sane" – *Robin Williams*

Madness is something we actually get driven into us as a youngster, the only problem is that 90% of the time we are taught that being 'mad' is a bad thing. When you look at the actual definition of madness two out of the three definitions in the dictionary are

'Extremely foolish behaviour'
'A state of wild or chaotic activity'

Is this not a good thing? Like is this not the thing we call 'fun' well, it's my method and this is what I class 'madness' as – FUN.

The definition of fun by the way 'behaviour or an activity that is intended purely for amusement and should not be interpreted as having any serious or malicious purpose' not much difference is there.

When I dive in with clients it is apparent that we are lacking time to ourselves, time for unplugging and having some mad time in our lives. I used to be the definition of this and the funny thing at the time is that I was seen as being in such amazing shape that my body would be what a lot of guys would actually love to have, abs all year round with veins popping out of my biceps I looked like one of those guys from 300 without the sprayed on six pack but let me really tell you about the amount of madness that went on in my life back then through my daily routine every single day, you tell me if it is 'fun' or not (note: I know you can't tell me, it was rhetorical, deal with it)

6am – wake – black coffee – no sweetener – 30 minutes cardio on treadmill in garage (even when it was mid-winter and below freezing)
7am – breakfast – oats, egg whites, veg
9am – work: desk job
11am – make an excuse to leave a meeting if I was in one to eat a meal but I would eat regardless – rice, chicken, veg plain
1pm – eat same meal again
3pm – oats, protein powder, banana
5pm – leave work for the gym
5:30pm – train for 2 hours
8pm – eat
8:30pm – prepare all my food for the next day
9:30pm – 20 minutes power walk on treadmill
10:00pm – shake and then bed

How much fun do you see in there?

Tell you what though, I was shredded, living with my mum and step-dad, I had all the girls wanting to look at me but no time for them, let me tell you this for free – there is NO way I would want to be back being that person when I know how much I have grown now.

If it was a non-work day I would be training in the morning and then taking my Tupperware to family get togethers, if I wasn't able to take my Tupperware then I wouldn't go, there would be an excuse and it would not be an option to stray off of my diet.

I have a task for you to do.

For the next week – and yes I want a week, not two or three days – write down every thing you do every 15 minutes in an excel sheet (I am happy to send mine if you want it ollie@revitalizationblueprint.com just drop me an email) from the moment you wake until the moment you go to bed, everything even if you spend 15 minutes taking a crap write 'toilet', write when you eat food, how long it takes to prepare it, the time it takes to drive to work, everything you can imagine it goes on there including the time you take scrolling and trolling on Facebook, pop it on. When it comes to the end of this I want you to go through each day (you can do it daily if it is easier) and highlight all the 15 minute blocks which you would consider 'fun' or time for you 'madness'.

The first time I done this it was an eye opener and it was for clients too, I've done it twice actually and the second time was to see how much time I was spending with specific money making activities when I was struggling with getting the funds I needed to pay all the bills when leaving the corporate world. I actually only had 60 minutes of fun over an entire 2 week period – in fact I put down 'training' as fun but in reality it wasn't so I took that out and there was a 60 minute fun period, that was watching a football match which was pre-recorded so I skipped over a lot of the 'boring' part. Another thing that jumped out at this time was that I took a long while to sleep, literally sitting in bed for an hour before I drifted off it seemed, waking for a piss 5 times a night (no, that is not normal no matter how much you justify it to yourself, once is too much).

So what did I do, how did I change?

I committed to myself what I was going to do, this was a time before I was married but I was still already with the future Mrs Matthews back then and I made sure I was accountable, during the week I would commit to one date night, this was not something I would ever be able to skip, Wednesday nights we done something we both wanted to do – Cinema, food, bowling, trampolining (we were the oldest in the venue but fuck it), trips to the beach, the thing I committed to here I found the hardest was to leave my phone at home or in the car glove box, that was scary but I figured that anyone who needed me in an emergency had the wife's number so could contact her if anything had to get through to me, anything else would wait, that goes for yourself too, NOBODY is that important I don't care if you have multiple businesses, multiple staff members or even multiple countries relying on you, if you can't take an evening off without dedicating yourself to the person you love most (after yourself) then your life is actually in a pretty fucked up state, sorry to say that but you are not that important, the world will not blow up if you turn your phone off for an hour, get over it.

Another thing is that I turned off and unplugged again at the weekend, yes ONE WHOLE DAY, one whole 24 hours where I couldn't be contacted and the way I done this was setting the guidelines with clients each time one would be set up and get on board, you know, even the clients paying me £5k/month and above will respect this – I get responses to messages within 12 hours on working days, the important wording being 'working days' and that includes UK public holidays too, that includes weekends, I state when we get working together than most of the time I will respond at weekends but not Sundays, most of the time I will respond in the evenings but not Wednesdays, set the markers and stick to them. I know what you're thinking here again – I work a 9-5 then I have to get home and sort the children out, do the house work, I am launching a business too in the evenings I haven't got time to have fun in my life....shut up! Gary Vee mentioned something which was 100% true and whilst you know me and I like to believe in health first there is a time we have to hypothetically 'hustle' but all that this requires is a little planning like this.

24 hours in a day
Working 9 to 5 = 16 hours left
Travel to and from work 2 hours max = 14 hours left
Sleep 6 hours minimum = 8 hours left
Play with children (this can be fun time too) 2 hours = 6 hours left
Time with the wife 2 hours = 4 hours left
Work on new business for 4 hours = 0 hours left

Be organised you have 4 hours of fun in here that is around 17% of your day for fun. It will hurt people the most who need the kick up the arse and I mean it with love, why? Because when I got told I needed to grow a pair of balls and be more organised in order to have more fun, more madness in my life what was my response? 'Fuck off, you don't know me' I had to learn the hard way and now I am proud to say I am pretty close – OK some weeks we all slip, guess what, it is called being human but 90% of the time I am on the ball with madness now.

8. Marriage

"When someone shows you who they are, believe them the first time." – *Maya Angelou*

People often get confused with the actual term 'marriage' and it's in there because it is much more than just a relationship between two human beings brought together by love and charged a ridiculous amount to pop a ring on the finger and have some bubbly with friends and family, yeah I simplified it a little but you get the picture, biggest advice for anyone getting married – set a budget at the start.

Marriage is about relationships, the relationships we encounter day in day out from the moment that we wake up to the moment we go to bed. The relationship with yourself, how do you want to be, how are you actually now and what can we do to fill that divide up. Relationships with your friends, which link into the madness portion, are you seeing your friends as much as you want and are they really your true friends. Remember what Jim Rohn famously said.

'You are the average of the five people you spend the most time with'

It couldn't be more to the point, so much truth within right there. When you look at the five people around you, the people you spend the most time with how do they make you feel when you are with them but more importantly, how do you feel in the couple of hours before you meet? Are you getting anxious? Are you feeling stressed? Are you feeling like you are going to be compromised in any particular way?

Let me tell you a story and you will be able to resonate with this, I guarantee it. You're reading this book because you're someone who wants to make a difference so you will probably have been exactly the same as I was with this type of guy. I had a friend who I had known for a while, we used to train for a while together and he actually helped me through one of the build ups for a previous show, good to have someone to spot and get you through when you really do feel like death warmed up. Now, it was all good for the first couple of years and then I would get him missing sessions, it isn't an issue if someone doesn't want to train but he would say he would be then and not turn up, I'd get a text saying he got held up at work or something, this happened regularly and it turned out he had some money issues and was trying to hide it. The conversations turned when we did meet up from being the good guy to hang around with it started becoming a stress for me to see him, not because I didn't want to but I just know that I would have to listen to every excuse under the sun as to the reasons why 1, he wasn't going to the gym (to be honest I couldn't care less if he trained or not, it's his choice) and 2, why he couldn't get the money together he needed to survive properly and even get to a job interview – I ended up loaning him a few hundred pounds to get a new suit and get to the job interview, he made another excuse as to why he couldn't get to the interview this time, I wasn't expecting to see that money again to be honest. I suddenly stopped hearing from him and a month after all this happened he then called me asking if wanted to grab a coffee, I got to the shop and I could tell he was expecting the coffees to be on me, not an issue at all really apart from the last 10 coffees were on me! In driving to this meet up I was having some stress issues and I knew within myself I had to cut this person off, I lost sleep the night before because I was getting worried about what excuse he was going to come up with, and, me being me, I would want to help him as that is what I do. He used to be one of the five closest people to me, this was 5 years ago, in the past 5 years since I cut him off I have grown ridiculously both in my own self and my business, it was no coincidence.

So write down a list, the five closest people to you, and then write down 3 postives and 3 negative each one adds to your life, the people you really should have close to you and who serve you as much as you serve them will jump out, why? Because you will find it easy to list the positives and bloody hard to list the negatives for these guys. The ones who you should cut off, they will also jump out, you will see why.

Here's the hard bit – I had to find a way to cut off some family members to personally grow and even start to reach my potential, that was hard at first but it didn't mean actually physically cutting them off all it meant was owning my mind within these relationships and it's something I dive into with clients more and more as time goes on. What do I mean? Well, don't take anything personally and make sure you are mindful of what you're speaking to them about I even had to do this with my own Mum, she will be one of the people reading it so 'Hi Mum! Love You! You better had brought your own copy!' but here's what happened.

When I was working a corporate job it was always classed as 'safe' you know even when you hear of redundancies left, right and centre the average Joe will always deem this contract to be 'safe', you rock up, do your work, log out and unplug at the end of the day, easy. Well when I left this world (after losing two management jobs 1st due to offshoring and 2nd due to budget cuts) I was going into the unknown for my mum, for her it didn't seem like I had a real job (wtf is a real job right?!) and every time I saw her she would always ask 'are you ok? Are you busy?' and the answer was always yes, I never got these questions when I was working a regular job, even when I was working in fitness they would never come and this used to frustrate me. I done some work on myself and realised I could cut off her beliefs, they aren't mine, I have no business in taking on board someone else's beliefs I can't control them I can only control my own so for this relationship to thrive I would have to do so, know I am successful and make sure I believed it 100% in actual fact it wasn't until mid way through 2017, after being in this industry for years, that she said 'you're like one of those Entrepreneur things' aren't you. She doesn't ask how I am doing that much now, she knows how well I am doing.

So this is where we get to the nitty gritty of relationships we have friends, we have family and we have our partners, the latter what people really think of when we say 'marriage' and usually it's what people focus on in order to 'be there for someone', I made this mistake in the year I got married, it wasn't that long ago and honestly I wasn't sure I should put it into this book but I promised to be 100% authentic and not hide anything, it is the biggest reason why my program The Revitalized Man has had so much success, because I AM REVITALIZED. In the run up to the wedding I noticed a bit of change in my wife to be, stress, illness and generally losing awareness in multiple areas, it is what happens when people become overwhelmed and I noticed it from when I had a bout of anxiety a few years back so I wanted to support, I took my foot off the gas with my health and with my business, I was allowed right? I was getting married, it was the most important day of my life. It was the worst decision I could ever make at that moment in time, the repercussions of taking my foot off the gas took a long while to fix.
The big day came and we made it, that was until the proofs came back with our photos, I had the biggest football face

(soccer for you crazy Americans) I could ever imagine, I had let my health and my weight slide, well, climb more than slide shall we say! I had 20 kilograms to lose and this was the kick up the arse I really needed, the problem was that it wasn't the only thing I let slide, I lost focus in the business and the money I made in the first few years of growing was good, the money I made in the year of getting married had dropped by around 40%, that wasn't good, in the year I needed to make more money than the previous years I had dropped a massive amount. I had the firework up my arse and I am happy to say that right now I have the things in place, I advise everybody to have a coach, I have three right at this moment and I will never ever forget to invest in myself again even for the lady who means the most to me in the entire world. Remember when you last went on an airplane? Well, they go through the safety briefing and tell you if shit hits the fan then fix your air mask first, because if you aren't strong enough yourself you can't help anyone around you. I forgot to fix my own mask first and as a result I couldn't even undo my seatbelt let alone go and help the people I wanted to help around me, don't make this mistake, invest in yourself for the good of the relationships with those closest to you.

That ties into the last relationship I want to briefly go over, the relationship with that dude staring right back at you when you look into the mirror, how can you serve this person better than any other person on this planet?

It takes a lot of courage to look at why you want to change and sometimes we want a six pack for the wrong reasons, I did if you remember my 'madness' chapter, it wasn't a nice thing, I had abs all year round and it wasn't good mentally for me to be in this situation, I mean, yes I went to the other extreme and it made me embarrassed but it was different, I wasn't embarrassed because other people thought I had got a bit cuddly, no, I was embarrassed because I had let myself down, I had cheated on the most important relationship I had in my life, the relationship with myself, it was like I had even gone and done the worst form of cheating in my opinion and gone and cheated on 'me' with multiple hookers, and I don't mean the expensive ones who play it off as escorts either!

So in wrapping up here I want you to really look into it.

Do the relationships in your life serve you?
Does the relationship you have with yourself serve you right now?
How would you change these relationships?
Within the next 12 months who have you got to get rid of in order to grow and start reaching your full potential?

This may hurt, it did with me.

9. Money

"Too many people spend money they earned..to buy things they don't want..to impress people that they don't like." -*Will Rogers*

Money is the route of all evil, apparently, but money is cool, we like money and we love working out ways to get more of it, this is one of the shortest chapters but it will make you think none the less. A lot of the thinking around money comes from when you have either a scarcity or abundance mindset and it usually determines what you attract into your life, not just with money but other things, love, happiness, health and so forth. What does this actually mean?

Well, let's start off with 'scarcity' – the state of being scarce or in short supply.

I was actually brought up in this world without my mum being aware of what she was kind of engraining into my brain, why? Because it was about being safe – don't push your luck and make sure you prepare because there is always a limited supply of things around the world. This was a limiting belief I used to live my life by and it was actually engrained into my mum by her mum, my nan who was brought up in the early 1920s around Norwich in what can only be said to be a poverty area, in fact, before my nan passed she was asked to share her stories of the time growing up in Norwich and I want to let you see where this world of scarcity was developed and passed on down the generations purely because of love and protection.

"We lived in a slum house, up Nicholls Yard in Barrack Street. There was about a dozen of us all had to use the same toilet, we had about one tap in the yard and we had an old washhouse in the yard with a big old coppel where my mother used to do the washing, up the corner there was a big old coppel, my father used to have to light that coppel with a lot of newspapers to get the coppel to boil, you know, and all that.
Well then I was ill with diptheorier and I had to go into the isolation hospital, I was about 5 years old. I went in there and I can remember crying all the while whilst I was there, although you was dressed and you was running about, you know, you was dressed and they used to let you run about but you weren't allowed out because of the infection. Well, anyhow, after I came out I went back to the house and my brother had got diptheorier, Billy, so he had to go back in where I had come out because that was infectious. Well anyhow they said, because we lived in these slums they would have to find us a better house because we only had one room downstairs, one big living room downstairs and one bedroom upstairs, in the bedroom my mother and father's bed used to be this side, Billy used to sleep at the foot of the bed at the top of the stairs Elsie and Ethel used to sleep in a three quarter bed that side of the room and I used to be up that corner in this hear crither fair thing, well anyway after a little while when Billy came out of the hospital they give us a new council house and it was like living in paradise because we got a toilet of our own,

a bathroom with a bath in it and a coppel where you used to have to boil the water to have a bath, we used to have to boil the water to have a bath, you know." – Gladys Courtnell (Norwich Memories)

You can see where the scarcity mindset came from within my family now right? Well, as we have spoken about you will have to choose, do you want to live your life by other people's beliefs or your own beliefs? That is the biggest question you will ever have to answer and also it will give you the most power when you do answer it.

Abundance – is this where you want to be?

' the situation in which there is more than enough of something'

This really is an ideal place to be right? You have a mindset set to abundance and you know you will be able to grow and always get more wealth, more health, more happiness because there is more than enough around the universe for it to go around. Cool right?

Well, it works with money, trust me but in order to get it to have the same effect it is not always money you need to focus on, get the balance right in the other 4 M's and you will be more than on the way to increasing your financial situation hell, I have had multiple guys more than double their income within the first month of being part of The Revitalized Man program using the Revitalization Blueprint.

Do you know where your money is going?

I was on the phone to a guy the other day, talking about the Revitalization Blueprint and how he can start to implement some of the things I talk about before actually working with me, why? Because he wasn't in a position there and then to be able to invest in himself the amount needed to get going. We said that in order to know what is needing to be saved we needed to know what is going out in the first place, and what is coming in so just like I do with clients when they sign up for the nutrition side of things and take a food diary for a week we said to take a money diary, know what you are spending every single penny on and you will get a lot more awareness, but you will also know you have places where you can gain money, patterns open up and you are able to notice them before they get to be a problem but even better, these patterns sometimes are opportunities to develop a world of abundance when it comes to money too.

So find out, are you living in a world of scarcity or abundance and decide if it is because of your beliefs or the beliefs you were brought up on, finally, if you need to, treat your bank account like your diet and get on board with a money diary, see exactly what is going on day to day even minute to minute.

See, it's not a long chapter, it doesn't have to be because money is simply a result of achieving balance in the other 4 M's, simple.

10. Moving Mountains – The Everest Obsession

'Accidents on big mountains happen when people's ambitions cloud their good judgment. Good climbing is about climbing with heart and with instinct, not ambition and pride.' – Bear Grylls

Why does this have it's own chapter and is not just thrown under the mindset side of things?

Well, it is more important to look at your journey, look at what you may face and what you have already faced head on, overcome and conquered than just looking into the mindset of why, and what you are doing.

Everest, Sagarmāthā as it is known in Nepal and Chomolungma in China the highest mountain on planet Earth. It may seem a bit off topic to be talking about this obsession of mine in a book aimed at YOUR body upgrade that we are doing one day at a time however this may be the most important chapter I write in this book, it certainly is more important to me with my clients than what they eat, how they exercise and how they go about their daily routine, I guarantee this.

Everest is a dream to many climbers, the highest point that many won't reach, the highest point in earth that many have tried to climb and their lives were taken by the mountain, the mountain which is a grave holding the bodies of the people she has conquered in her arms as other climbers walk past, one-step-at-a-time. 29035 feet high no man made machine can put you there, you have to go there yourself. From the first documented attempt under the leadership of Charles Howard-Bury in 1921 to the first person, along with his Sherpa Tenzing Norgay, to reach the peak Sir Edmund Hillary exactly 64 years ago to the day of myself writing this chapter (29th May 1953), since then many more have tried and over 290 people have lost their lives in the process, Brits that have conquered Everest include legends and idols of mine such as Bear Grylls and Sir Ranulph Fiennes who was allowed by the mountain to conquer her at 65 years old, there is a certain way people have to go about this mountain, this unprecedented task ahead of them and this is what it has to do with your health.

Everest is made up of 5 camps sitting at different altitudes which all need to be adapted by the body to be able to survive at:-

- Base camp 17500ft
- Camp 1 19685ft
- Camp 2 21000ft
- Camp 3 23625ft
- Camp 4 26085ft
- Summit 29035ft

When a climber embarks on the task of climbing Everest they have to go to base camp, spend time there to acclimatise before then climbing to camp 1, at camp 1 they will spend a night or two to acclimatise before dropping down to base camp again, the body isn't designed to be at these heights for a long time and especially if they aren't acclimatised to it, they need to adapt. Then they go up to camp 1, then to camp 2 depending on the time, acclimatise and drop down to base camp, they repeat the process, up to camp 1, through to 2 and up to 3, acclimatise and back down, finally they do the same up to camp 4 (some climbers have been known to miss the acclimatisation at 4 which is a risky process with camp 4 and above named 'The Death Zone'. Finally they drop to base camp, recover for a couple of weeks before climbing through all the camps and up to the summit.

What does this have to do with your own journey, your own health?

It is never linear when you are here, but you do have to start, it all starts with an idea 'I want to get healthy' this idea has motivation 'I hate how I look', 'I want to provide for my family more', 'I want more money' and so on. The idea for these climbers was to get to the summit AND return down safely. That is actually the idea when we have our own health to think about too. We have to first off climb up to base camp, 17500 feet, this is typically an 8 day trek to get to (4 to return down). This is usually the hardest step but everyone needs to take it, one foot in front of the other, one step at a time. The problem is, that even people who have quick fixes need to get this step underway but they try to get up the mountain in one go they trek the 8 days to base camp and then proceed to climb the mountain without stopping at base camp, without stopping at any camp on the way, without acclimatising and usually without any food OR oxygen, they don't make it, they fall into an open crevasse or get taken out by an avalanche and usually if they somehow survive will quit and that will be the end of the attempt on health, until the next quick fix is handed their way.

So my moving mountains analogy is this – you will have to come back down to go back up but consistency is where you will get your results, consistency will allow you to reach the summit and keeping that consistency will allow you to get back to base camp without losing that health and actually be at a level you're able to thrive and build every day, one day at a time in your body upgrade.

Many people forget about the up and down process, I don't mean yo-yo dieting here, the true process we have call 'life' it happens to all of us. Let me describe my own journey here from the corporate world.

When I lost my second secondment due to off-shoring I was rock bottom but I knew I had to make a first step for anything to happen, this was the hardest step. I would literally wake up in the middle of the night screaming, get lots of sleep paralysis and have dreams of running away but getting stuck in the mud in the process. With me having been in the fitness industry before I was in the corporate world I was still scared of getting back in and earning as little money as before, even though it was, and still is, my passion. I had to believe, envision (remember those visualisation techniques they are so powerful) and make a plan to get out of the world I was in and trek to base camp (in my mind this was where I was no longer depressed whilst earning enough to support both my wife and I without having to answer to a 9 to 5 role). I actually remember a morning where it all changed, I was going to a seminar with two good friends, I had no money but these guys John Chapman and Leon Bustin allowed me to grab a lift to London for the seminar for free (they are two amazing YouTube stars now 'The Lean Machines') at the event in London I was given a ticket by the hosts 'Cliff and Marta Wilde' little did I know the inspiration would start here for my biggest journey ever, this was my first step to leaving the corporate world and essentially, my trek to base camp was underway.

That's what I mean by finding the kick that gets you to trek to base camp and when you're there being prepared to climb a camp but also return to the level again, here's the example: Someone, yourself even, may look to get in shape for their holiday, that requires them travelling to base camp (the first step) then going hard for their holiday up to camp 1, they stay there (first few days of holiday) then climb down (last part of the holiday when they may have lost a little shape BUT they've loved it so much it doesn't matter) the mistake people make here is that they end up going down trekking back home from base camp now, they've already acclimatised and their body knows what it's like to be where they wanted to be a week or two ago, if they stay at base camp (much further than where they started) then they will be able to get in better shape both physically and mentally staying acclimatised ready to get up to camp 2, rather than next year they have to make that long 8 day trip to base camp again THEN climb the FIRST camp and only end up where they were IF they didn't fall of the last time, consistency is so key here.

What I say to clients with this theory is that you cannot continue on the same path forever, sometimes we need to back track before we can progress higher, another example here:
You're doing to well, you've gotten to a habit and have trained real well with your One Day Body Upgrade for 28 days, you're spot on, feel amazing, stronger and have more energy all around, not only this you actually have increased your earnings in this time by 10%, then you get ill, you have a bout of the flu and you have to jump off of camp 2, where to? Base camp. Now it's knowing that coming down will make you better, your body will improve and recover on the way down and staying at base camp is enough to keep you ticking over whilst

you're ill, what happens to some people though? They use this illness to go back and take a trek back home 17500 feet lower than base camp which takes 4 days to get back this essentially means that they fall off on their nutrition along with their training, their meditation stops and basically they are a very limited version of the person they need to be and were a couple days ago when they were all acclimatised on camp 2, there is a long way back now, if someone even wanted to get back they now have to trek 8 days (not the 4 it took to get them back home) back to base camp before acclimatising at camp 1, coming down and then up to camp 2, all because they let their flu hit them so far, feeling sorry for themselves, binged out and stopped doing that they know they could do, consistency.

So know that life will happen, people say they don't get ill, I know people who haven't been ill for years it does happen and a lot is that when their body is under stress they never fall off of basecamp, they never drop past the point they were at before the last push up in their journey. The mind is so powerful here.

What all good climbers have in common is that they will know when to also turn back, they will know then the camp is a little out of reach and the summit needs a bit more consistency as the gap in weather isn't long enough to reach it, but they stay consistent, they stay moving forwards, going up or going down they still move forward. And that's exactly what you need to be aware of, a goal may not be able to be reached today it may need to turn back, check the sat nav, add a diversion and attempted again tomorrow or the next day, but consistency will keep you where you need to be and where you will be able to achieve that goal in the long term.

This is where people fall off the hypothetical mountain, they don't plan for set backs, they don't plan for life to happen and psychologically we absolutely hate it when we set a goal and fail, that is where the goal setting we spoke about earlier in the mindset chapter comes into play. Realise what you are aiming for, why you're aiming for it and what will happen both if you don't do it along with if you do make it happen, the truth can sometimes hurt but be so damn needed sometimes.

So to recap, don't expect your journey to be linear, there will be ups and downs but always realise how far you have come along the line and when you do go back down – make sure you don't leave base camp, the place way ahead of where you started, unless you want to start from scratch once again.

11. Putting It All Together

'You see something, then it clicks with something else, and it will make a story. But you never know when it's going to happen.' Stephen King

We have the plan, you are ready to put it all together and really upgrade, you know, your One Day Body Upgrade. I keep mentioning the title and there is a reason, we get it into our heads that something will be hard but in reality if we think about it as one day at a time, one step, one movement then you really do create epic shifts with ease, you flow from one state into the other without any stress.

Here we will go through the basics again keeping it so simple that you can even outsource preparation for someone else to do, just get them to read this book.

The Perfect Day

Now everybody will be different but I am going to go through what I envisaged to be my perfect day before I got into the full time world of being a fitness entrepreneur. Yours may be a little different and the timings may change too but what is important is that you write down what your perfect day looks like and when you want to get there by, this will be crucial to the accountability in getting you there and it is so much easier to know what 'perfect' looks like if you have imagined it in your head. Goals are everything.

6:30am
Wake up and grab some lemon squeezed into fresh room temperature water – great way to start the day, great for kidney and liver function which in turn will set your body up right to kick out the toxins which have built up from the day before.

Meditate and spend some time on my journal.

8:00am
Cardio session, nothing drastic but just to get the blood flowing, increase the heart rate, maybe on the spin bike maybe a steady jog outside, then walk the dogs.

9:00am
Breakfast
This would consist of something like oatmeal, almond milk and peanut butter with some fresh lemon in water again along with a bit of protein from a shake.

10:00am
Client meeting
I like to, if possible, meet up with my clients face to face, this may mean sometimes I will have to travel but it is something I take very seriously as in face to face contact you get a certain

interaction you cannot do via email. If we cannot meet up every week I will make sure this is a Skype conversation and that we will have the camera on in order to see facial expressions and gestures throughout the call.

12:00noon
Get back and walk the dogs for a short walk and follow this with lunch.
Lunch will be a salad of some sort, a meat source and carbohydrate as my main training session will come in the afternoon after another meeting.

2:00pm
Client meeting
As mentioned above this will ideally be face to face if not again I will take this on Skype with the camera on. I find that regardless of if you work from home and not just because of the interaction you get with the video call functions, Skype allows you to take a bit more pride in your appearance again which is something I feel is very important in the line of work we are in.

3:00pm
Snack
Something like some nuts, fruit and a protein shake – nothing that will take a long while to prepare but something which will fuel me for a workout.

4:00pm
Admin work – when I say admin work I am talking about doing my social media posts, any videos I need to record and emails I may need to personally make. My VA will take care of a lot of the administration items that come into my inbox.

5:00pm
Training session – this will involve weight training and some high intensity work, even someone like myself who has a big history and makes a living from fitness I don't want to be in the gym all evening I want to get home for my family and chill out.

7:00pm
Evening meal with family
I will always aim to have something pretty similar to the wife and family even if it means having something without sauce when they are having something but I pride myself in being able to have this time with the family where we won't talk about specific business items but we will appreciate each other's time and company.

8:00pm
Chill with the wife – date night or watch a film

9:30pm
Read for a little while in bed after completing my journal and lights out around 10:00pm roughly.

This routine is something I pride myself on, I wrote it when I had a full time job in the corporate world and visualised every part of it until the perfect day become more and more real and it wasn't a dream but actual reality.

The Perfect Day OUT

Life gets in the way sometimes right? You have meetings and as I mentioned above, I like to get to face to face meeting with clients so it is vital I put in this book some things to make sure you do in order to stick to good fuel and habits when travelling.

First things first, leave plenty of time, if it takes 3 hours to get somewhere then allow for 4 hours, sounds a bit silly, a whole extra 60 minutes but we will be stopping to get some steps up and here's a couple habits I make sure I do when going out for the day.

I always make sure I have at least 3 good meals ready in a cool bag, I may not have them but I damn sure know that if shit hit the fan and I got stuck at a services with hardly any healthy options then I would be covered.

I will make sure that I stop every 60-90 minutes for 15 minutes break and walk around, I make sure I rack up more steps with the habit we learnt earlier in the book and park the furthest away from the entrance to any services and when I come back I will walk the long way round back to the car too.

Inevitably you're going to have to have a coffee or a drink with a client and if you aren't able to deal with more water then the occasional diet soda will be ok buyt make sure you fuel when you get back on the journey home, get the hydration in there it is so important. When you are at the meeting if you are in a food place then look at healthier options on the menu, salads without the dressings, vegetables instead of fries and simple whole food ingredients, it is easy to stick to just be strong, you don't always need those nachos coated in cheese and pulled beef strips.

We're All Going On A Summer Holiday (Or Winter Trip)

We have these times in our lives where we have to let it all hang out, vacations are simply that, chill time, time for spending with loved ones and you know what, screw it, I will enjoy my vacation as I have earned every minute of it! You do not need to go out an binge but I can guarantee you paid a good amount of money for the trip so why not enjoy it. Chances are you have 2-4 weeks maybe of holidays a year if you are in a 'real' job so if you look at it it's like 2-3% of the year you're away. Maybe add another week for national holiday time and birthday (kill two birds with one stone, just be born on Christmas day, simple!) now that 3, let's say 5% of time maximum is not going to break the bank, just be an adult about it, you don't need to binge out every night, you are not so stressed you need to down a bottle of vodka each hour of the day because it is all inclusive, yes you have paid for the privilege, but you are an adult, if the goal of having an amazing life, amazing health and being able to provide for your family means a hell of a lot to you then you will be able to abide by this, trust me. And if you can't, you really aren't ready to be upgraded.

Family time

This is different from your vacation and national holidays this is time you spend dedicated to your family, inevitably you're going to be offered the left overs from your 3 year old's plate, I get that but you can easily help this by ordering a little less yourself. Enjoy the family time, this is time to be cherished and why you work so hard, not just in the board room but also in the gym, on the field, running the streets and in the kitchen. If you are an adult about life when it is time to be an adult then the family time will be time for you to chill, let your hair down (what's left of it!) and have some fun. Add this to the holiday time and you're looking about 10% of the time you're off your diet, this leaves 90% of the time to make sure everything is on point, I aim for 80% compliance with clients in order to get results, see where I am going with this?

12. The Small Stuff For Big Results

'Success in life is founded upon attention to the small things rather than to the large things; to the every day things nearest to us rather than to the things that are remote and uncommon.' – Booker T. Washington

So we have been through the things you should eat but it isn't always those three macros that make the most of difference in your everyday health. Here we will go through the small things, those little things that add up and are also in our food and lifestyle which make the biggest of impact.

You will learn the bits that will make the most difference to each of your One Day Body upgrades. Things like how you digest your food and why this is so important to not just being upgraded but feeling upgraded too, how stress can impact your upgrade and what to do in order to make sure it doesn't stop you, and the hormonal parts of our bodies which can be effected by what we eat and drink on a daily basis.

Let's begin…

Gut Health & Digestion

This is one of the biggest secrets of having a carefree feel good lifestyle right now, your gut, after all what is the point in putting so much amazing food into your body if you can't get the goodness out of it?

Your gut will allow you to digest the nutrients from the food, make use of the carbohydrates, the proteins and the fats in those food items. It is here that something called 'serotonin' is mainly produced in the body. Serotonin is a neurotransmitter and it is responsible for things we take for granted everyday, feel good factors such as your mood, sleep, appetite. Basically it is produced in the gut and needs to get to the brain, in doing so it will make sure you produce a major feel good factor and positivity will just seep out of you. If you don't eat good food and you go for the processed route a lot of the time with junk food then you are risking having digestive issues, putting the gut under unnecessary stress and basically stopping it from doing it's job and producing that serotonin, not only this but if you don't produce enough serotonin then you risk some dodgy toilet issues from one extreme to the other.

Stress

We live in a world of stress from the moment we wake up to the moment we go to bed we don't get away from stress. You have stress everywhere, addictions left, right and centre to social media mean that you don't just have your own stress but you see everyone else's problems too, more stress.

You wake up and are tired, stressed you have to go to work and you're late, you get to work and your employees haven't done the quality of work you expect of them, more stress. You finish work and the Mrs has had a moan that you have done something wrong, more stress so you need to take it out on something, you go to the gym, do some sprints, lift some weights, hit the bag but you are then fighting your stress with, you guessed it, more stress the cycle continues and it is vicious.
Add stress to the serotonin production in the gut, now we are designed to survive and that age old fight or flight syndrome kicks in, the body fires up it's adrenaline signals wanting to fight when we stress ourselves out, your body takes blood from the gut, we don't need to digest then we're about to fight after all, and your digestion quality does way down purely because of that big S word 'Stress'.

But as said we live in a world of stress and as long as you're aware of it there are things you are able to do. We can't go into much detail as it will add a hell of a lot to this book but certain things as taking 'me time', meditating, reading books to get away from things, sleeping with better quality, we will get to the sleep bit next.

All these things will allow you to handle stress and in actual fact, there is no such thing as a bad situation or stressful situation it is simply just how we perceive it.

Stress will tire you out I guarantee it, why? Because you won't digest food properly, meaning you won't get the energy from your food. You won't recover from the training you are doing and that will just add insult to injury when it comes to sleeping.

Sleep

This sounds pretty easy to do right? You lay down, close your eyes and off you go into dream world. But there is more to it than that.
When we sleep we have 5 different stages that we go in and out of during the night 1,2,3,4 and REM (rapid eye movement) sleep. We go in and out of a cycle from 1 to REM throughout the night beginning with shorter periods in REM and gradually they become longer.

Stage 1 – Can be awoken pretty easily and sometimes you may experience that falling sensation which wakes you up right here.

Stage 2 – This is where you won't move your eyes too much and your brain waves slow down too.

Stage 3 – Really slow brain waves now and not much movement.

Stage 4 – Slow waves called delta waves are produced here. 3 and 4 are deep sleep.

Stage 5 – REM – breathing becomes more rapid, eyes move rapidly, limb muscles kind of get paralysed, increased heart rate, increased blood pressure and us blokes may even get that good old 'morning wood' feeling right here. You dream mostly in this stage of sleep and if you get woken up here then you will more than likely remember your dreams.

Your body will go through multiple cycles of the sleep patterns in the night and getting the deep sleep will help you recover and feel refreshed the next morning.

There is a problem though, to get into a good sleep pattern this doesn't just start with when your head hits the pillow but rather a good hour or so beforehand certain habits are good to take on board such as:

- Turn off electronic items even off of stand by – these produce a blue light which is what the sun gives out and signals the brain to wake up, this does mean turning the phones off and laptops off before bed.
- Read a good book which isn't business focused and really switch yourself off.

- And probably my favourite – sex, this will help, not sure if any studies say so but I like it before bed and it's my book so it is going in there.

If we don't get adequate sleep then you are setting yourself up to really need those coffee's the next day so this is one of the most important 'small things' here in this chapter.

Hydration

Our bodies are made up of around 55-65% water, pretty much shows how important it is to make sure you get enough of it per day to replenish what we use in our everyday lives both in sweat and respiration. Even a 5% drop in hydration can results in massive performance decreases and I don't just mean in the gym or on the sports field but in the board room too, your brain function will dramatically decrease, your attention span will go majorly down, your focus will be next to zero and you basically will not be able to upgrade your body the way you really want to.
So, how do we aim to sort this? Well, in the food you eat inevitably you will be getting some levels of hydration throughout and this will help but you will need to be drinking fluids throughout the day to make sure you are fully hydrated. Getting about 3 litres of water into you throughout is a good start building it up by having water with meals (some people

will say this isn't great for digestion but I believe it is a good place to be mindful of getting the fluid in there) have a bottle of water with you when you're working and sip on it as much as you can, if this is an issue then just simply set an alarm every 30 minutes or something roughly in good intervals to have a glass of water, if you are working out then have another 500ml for every hour at least, more if possible, you can't really overdo it unless you are drinking copious amounts like 10+ litres per day without sweating much, if you did this you would be potentially setting yourself up for something called hypaneutremia which is when you dilute your blood sodium levels and this could become fatal, so don't do that, please.

Remember, you will also get fluid from coffee and tea if you have them so these will be a little bonus on top, again if people say the caffeine in them is a diuretic then they are right in a way but the ratio of caffeine to water will really make this effect on the body pretty much zero.

Vitamins and Minerals. (pics need to be from stock images royalty free)

We hear something every day on balanced diet, essential nutrient dense foods and sufficient macronutrient profiling for our energy expenditure. But what about our micronutrient profile – our Vitamins and Minerals that are essential for our body to work and perform the way they do! This article will give you the low down on what they are and how they help your body function.

What are Vitamins and Minerals?

In simple terms they are essential nutrients that the body requires in small amounts to work efficiently and can be obtained from a varied and balanced diet. The body requires recommended daily allowances (see tables) to allow it to perform sufficiently. Because the body works the same, whether you are an athlete or a non-athlete, the micronutrient profile remains the same. Later in the article I will discuss when the recommended allowances may need to increase.

Vitamins

There are 2 types of vitamins that the body requires and I am going to spend some time explaining them and how they work within the body...

- Fat soluble vitamins

These vitamins are found in fatty foods eg, animal fats, oils, dairy liver, oily fish. They can be stored within the body in the liver and fatty tissues for future use; therefore it is not necessary to eat foods containing them every day.

The following table will show you the different fat soluble vitamins and their involvement within the body:

NAME	FUNCTION	SOURCE	RDA*
Vitamin A	strengthen immunity; help vision; keep skin healthy	cheese, eggs, fortified low fat spreads, yogurt	0.7mg men 0.6mg women
Vitamin D	helps regulate calcium and phosphate in the body	sunlight, oily fish, fortified fat spreads, breakfast cereal, powdered milk	Body takes what it needs mainly from primary source of sunlight
Vitamin E	helps maintain cell structure by protecting cell membranes	plant oils, nuts, seeds, wheat germ	4mg men 3mg women
Vitamin K	needed for wounds to heal (clots blood)	green leafy veg, veg oils, cereals	0.0001mg/kg of body weight

RDA – recommended daily amount to be taken daily
- Water soluble vitamins

These vitamins are found within fruits, vegetables and grains. They cannot be stored within the body and are therefore required on a daily basis. If you have more than your body requires then you will expel the extra when you urinate. These vitamins can be destroyed by heat or exposure to the air so it is worth noting that many vitamins are lost in the surrounding water when using the food for cooking, eg boiling. Better to steam or grill to keep the vitamins within the source of food you are preparing

The following table shows you the water soluble vitamins and their involvement within the body:

NAME	FUNCTION	SOURCE	RDA
Vitamin C	protects cells; maintains connective tissue; heals wounds	oranges, red/green peppers, strawberries, blackcurrants, broccoli, Brussel sprouts, potatoes	40mg per day for adults
Vitamin B1 - Thiamin	releases energy from food by helping break it down; keeps nerves and muscle tissue healthy	vegetables, peas, fresh & dried fruit, eggs, breads, cereals, liver	1mg men 0.8mg women
Vitamin B2 - Riboflavin	keeps skin, eyes & nervous system healthy; helps release energy from carbohydrates	milk, eggs, fortified cereals, rice (note – UV can destroy this vitamin so keep food sources out of direct sunlight)	1.3mg men 1.1mg women
Vitamin B3 - Niacin	produces energy from foods; keeps nervous and digestive systems healthy	meat, fish, wheat flour, maize flour, eggs, milk	17mg men 13mg women
Pantothenic Acid	helps release energy from the food we eat	all meat and veg, cereals, whole grains, porridge, eggs	amounts needed will be obtained from the diet
Vitamin B6 -	allows body to use	variety of foods;	1.4mg men

Pyridoxine	and store protein and carbohydrates; helps haemoglobin (the substance that carries o2 around the body)	pork, poultry, fish, bread, whole cereals, eggs, vegetables, soya beans, peanuts, milk, potatoes	1.2mg women
Folic Acid	works with B12 to form healthy blood cells; reduces risks of central nervous system defects in unborn babies	broccoli, Brussel sprouts, liver, spinach, asparagus, peas, chickpeas, brown rice, cereals	Adults require 0.2mg
Vitamin B12	makes red blood cells; releases energy from food	meat, salmon, cod, milk, cheese, eggs, cereals	0.0015mg per day for adults (note- vegan would need supplement)

Minerals

Now we have covered vitamins it seems only fair to cover minerals in the same way, as they are equally as important! Minerals are needed by our body to help us build strong teeth and bones. They also control body fluids inside and outside of cells. Another main function is that they can turn the food you eat to energy.

There are 2 main essential minerals required by our body and the following table will explain their functions in more detail:

NAME	FUNCTION	SOURCE	RDA
Calcium	helps to build strong teeth and bones; regulates muscle contraction, including the heartbeat; ensures blood clots	milk, cheese, dairy, green leafy, veg, soya beans, tofu, soya drinks, nuts, bread, fish where you eat the bones (sardines)	Adults require 700mg per day
Iron	helps make red blood cells, which carry o2 around the body	liver, meat, beans, nuts, dried fruit, wholegrains, cereals, soybean flour, dark-green leafy veg (note – liver not to be eaten if pregnant as rich in vitamin A which can damage an unborn baby)	8.7mg men 14.8mg women

That has covered some of the more common vitamins and minerals that make up your requirements for a healthy micronutrient profile. There are many other substances that are also required to make up a healthy diet but all are found in your daily diet.

Here is a simple picture of a food guide pyramid that shows you the amounts of food you should be eating per day. This is to ensure nutrient dense foods are met:

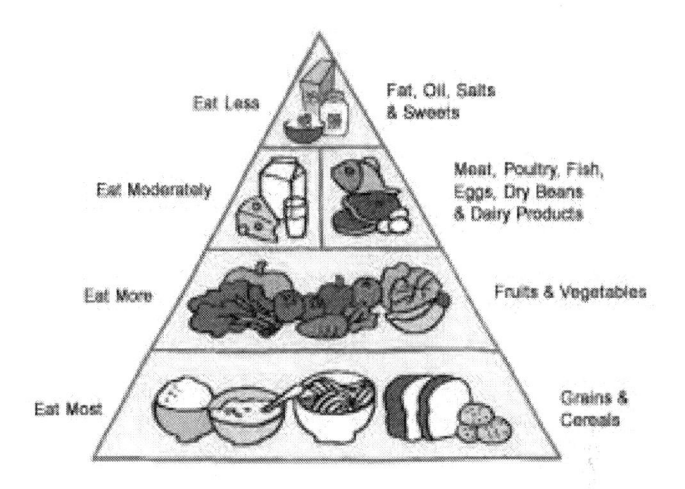

Food Pyramid:
- Eat Less: Fat, Oil, Salts & Sweets
- Eat Moderately: Meat, Poultry, Fish, Eggs, Dry Beans & Dairy Products
- Eat More: Fruits & Vegetables
- Eat Most: Grains & Cereals

Now that I have discussed how vitamins and minerals function in the body, I just want to touch base on the difference in the amount that elite and performance athletes may require due to the demands on their body:

As we know, exercise stresses many metabolic pathways in the human body. When an athlete exercises, the demands for micronutrients also increases due to muscle biochemical adaptation; essentially exercise increases turnover and loss of micronutrients. The energy intake for an athlete is also far greater than that of an average human, sometimes their daily menu being 2/3s greater than that of a sedentary individual, so in turn the RDA of a performance athlete would need to be increased, not to mention the need for muscle building, repair and maintenance of lean body mass. It should also be noted that if an athlete trains indoors, ie gymnasts, figure skaters etc, then the need for Vitamin D supplementation may be required as they will have minimal contact with direct sunlight and possibly a poor vitamin D status.

Who is at risk from not reaching their daily recommended allowance of vitamins and minerals?

In the majority of cases we can easily hit our targets of micronutrients by just eating a good nutrient dense diet daily but there are a few groups of people who may be required to take supplementation:

- Those who restrict calorie intake, ie a body builder cutting for a contest
- Have severe weight loss practices
- Those who eliminate one or more food group, ie vegans, vegetarians etc
- Those who consume unbalanced diets

If you feel you are possibly in one of the above categories then I would advise to seek out further guidance as to whether you should be supplementing your diet.

Cholesterol

'I have high cholesterol' this is something we have pretty much heard regularly from one person or another, the problem that a lot of doctors set us up with is that they test first off for what we call 'total cholesterol' which is a total sum of both 'good' and 'bad' cholesterol.

Not knowing the total LDL (bad) and total HDL (good) is like knowing that there were six goals in a football match but you don't know if it was 5-1 or 3-3, two very different outcomes.

So what I recommend for people to do is that if they're getting their cholesterol levels checked is to make sure that they get a full test done and find out their total LDL and total HDL so that you can get a good look at the bigger picture. Cholesterol is seemingly looked at as a bad thing but in reality we need cholesterol to survive and we need it in our diet from sources such as good fats and red meat along with egg yolks. I will put a good amount of money that you will not get high BAD cholesterol levels by eating good healthy food, it is a sedentary lifestyle, high stress levels (when not managed), poor diet filled with junk food and processed food, alcohol and smoking that will make the biggest impact on increasing your LDL levels.

Supplements

Lastly in this chapter I want to go through the cherry on the top, supplements.

Here are 4 supplements I recommend to clients to make sure they're at the top of their health for the day of awesomeness that is ahead of them.

1. Multivitamins

As well as getting your vitamins through the food you eat a multivitamin supplement is a major boost to your diet. By eating the correct amount of protein, carbs and fats each meal you will get plenty of vitamins each day.
With that said, the reality is we are all getting busier every day. There is a lot more distractions and time can be limited. So if the odd meal is missed or you have a day not quite up to your usual standards, a multivitamin supplement will help you avoid vitamin deficiencies. This is vitally important if you are serious about increasing your endurance and strength.

How much do you need?
Usually you will only need to take one per day, preferably with a meal.

Other benefits include..
Better sleep - Zinc helps to get better quality sleep.
Less illness - Vitamin c helps your immune system.
Faster recovery - Calcium and iron help faster recovery from strength training.

2. Fish oil

Taking an omega-3 supplement is a huge boost to your diet and will help you achieve better results. This supplement has been popular amongst those wanting to increase endurance and strength for a long time now. There are a lot of other benefits too including..

Reduced inflammation - less injuries etc

Decreased body fat - fish oil helps to burn fat.
Less soreness - reduced soreness from strength training
Increased muscle and heart health.

Ideally you want to be eating fish with good amounts of omega-3 several times a week. Still by taking the supplement as well it will keep you topped up and help avoid deficiencies.

How much do you need?
Usually one capsule per day or 1 tsp per day of the liquid version. Everyone has a different preference for when to take it, I find it can work well soon after your workout to help reduce muscle soreness.

3. Creatine

If you're wanting to build your mental clarity and focus, creatine is another essential supplement for you. It works well for explosive and high intensity exercise so perfect to sprint past someone on the run or bike. Exactly what is required from your workouts if you want to build endurance and strength. However you want to make sure you take a good quality one and I recommend using one without needing a loading phase. A poor quality creatine supplement can leave you feeling bloated and often not feeling any effect on your workout.

Creatine monohydrate in powder form works best.

How much do you need?
Again this varies person to person but usually taking one scooped dose up to an hour before you train works very well. (This is if you're using the monohydrate powder form). It can have a major positive impact on your workouts if you take it pre-workout and set you up nicely especially in your effort sessions. Some people take it post-workout and claim this helps their recovery too.

4. Whey protein powder

Here it is, the most common and known supplement for pretty much the entire fitness industy. The protein shake. I tend to avoid protein bars as they are mostly full of sugar and other chemicals. A good quality whey protein powder can be very beneficial to your training for endurance and strength, perfect to enhance recovery for your next hard session.

Protein should of course be consumed evenly throughout the day via your meals. You need it to repair and maintain your muscles especially when you're training at a higher intensity. But realistically a protein shake offers many other benefits..

It's quick and easy. You can take it about with you. Have one before or after your workout. Some people have one before AND after. It also means you can get the protein as soon as you want/ need it. That's a big bonus there.
One scoop is usually around 25 grams of protein so that's right up there with your other high protein foods.

It can also be quite good value if you shop around. Look on the Internet for good deals but make sure it's 100% safe.

How much do you need?
Some people like to have 1-2 per day depending on their goals. Others have 3-4. As long as you are getting protein from the foods you eat you should be able to integrate the shakes into your day to suit your lifestyle.
Commonly they work well in the morning, before or after a workout and before bed.
Take one scoop (25g) each shake and that should see you get the benefits.

The small stuff is actually ironically one of the most important pieces in this book, but don't worry, although there is a bit of science in here I will take all of the boring stuff out of the mix in the final chapters and show you how to put it all together at once in an easy One Day Upgrade style.

Here you know what supplements to take, when to take them, why to take them, what nutrients are needed both micro and macro and just overall how to be totally awesome with your upgrade.

13. The Three Phases

"The path to success is to take massive, determined action" – Anthony Robbins

This should be at the start right? Wrong, if I had put the three phases of how to complete the Revitalization Blueprint at the start chances are most people would have skipped and just started going in full speed essentially blind, here is where is should be, it's correct place, near to the end just before you put it all together.

The Revitalization Blueprint is broken down into three phases, each one vital in your journey towards success and what is so important is that you don't look at it as 3 phases and you're done but rather 3 phases and you can continue to cycle and grow each and every time you complete the Blueprint.

Phase 1 – Align
Phase 2 – Design
Phase 3 – Refine

Each one will take a different amount of time depending on the person's goal but I am going to go through each phase individually right now and show you why each is needed and why you should really deep dive into the short term goals you decide upon within each phase.

Phase 1 – Align

Alignment is crucial, if you aren't aligned to what you want to achieve it can seem a chore rather than a journey towards fulfilment and 100% Revitalization, alignment shows us what you are not just able to achieve but more what you are willing to achieve throughout the time you are working on your own self.

When I take a client on board after we have had initial talks and agree that they are the client who I want to work with along with myself being the coach that they want to have help them we will look at their goals with something I like to call my 'Triple H Method' (I was a wrestling fan!)

How Long – have you got to achieve it
How Much – do you have to change/lose/gain/earn
How Come – you want to change/lose/gain/earn

If these are in line you are already looking towards a successful journey here, if you set yourself too short a time frame then you set yourself up for failure, if you set yourself too little or too much of the 'how much' you are setting yourself up for failure and the 'how come' is when you know you are doing it for YOU and nobody else.

The align phase will get these goals on paper, short, medium and long term and we will set the path, usually if someone is wanting to gain muscle before revealing their physique then the align phase is the building phase but it is not just about building muscle it is also about setting the agreement with the inner self in order to build habits, build commitment and build up routine which you are then able to take on board for the following two phases. I would say 8-12 weeks is a good marker here for the first 'align' phase.

After the end of the 12 weeks there is a full evaluation of the wins along with the lessons learned throughout, what has gone well, what has gone poorly and we make sure that we take these learning's on board for the following phases.

Phase 2 – Design

We have already designed this right? Wrong, let's look at what is really involved when we design.

We have the foundations built right now from the first 'align' phase and now it is time to lay the supporting walls followed by the water tight roofing at the end, what does this mean for you exactly? Well, in the example of the first align phase we said about building muscle, it is now time to push and reveal that muscle to yourself when looking in the mirror. Fitness will be stepped up, you have been laying the foundations now it is time to increase and get even fitter, focus will be stepped up too, remember I had people double their earnings in the first month? Well, this is now going to be 3-4 months in, I will let you do the math.

Time moves on and sometimes our goals change too so we will set more short term goals in this phase using the 'Triple H' method once again and we know we will be achieving them goals, guaranteed. It is here we use the discipline built up in the 'align' phase to really design the life you want, we will look deeper in relationships you have with people around you, relationships with yourself, how is the money situation looking, how much fun are you actually having? How strong is your mind right now along with how much has it developed?

This phase again could be another 8-12 weeks, maybe more, every person is an individual and has individual goals, I don't do 'cookie cutter'.

Following this phase we evaluate once again, we define the successes you've had, the hurdles you have managed to overcome and the overall journey you have been on and how it has matched up with the Blueprint of your life.

Phase 3 – Refine

Ever done a diet, dropped a hell of a lot of weight only to stop and have it return again? This is where that stops, I will not have a client go through this because I don't believe in 'diets' I believe in sustainability via changing habits and building lives.

Phase 3 is where we kind of reset the body, you see, over time the body gets used to a state of homeostasis, it's 'set point' so to speak and it likes being there, this is why you can usually drop holiday weight pretty quickly, you go on holiday at 80kg, return at 84kg and 2 weeks later without dieting you're back to 80kg, this is the place the body can sit without a lot of stress, it likes this place. Now we have to aim to reset the body's point of homeostasis and in doing this we kind of balance at the position we are now at. So if you've dropped 10kg (22lb) you will then aim to stay at this for 6-8 weeks, yes I know, you want to keep pushing but this is long term, let's set a new start point and enjoy life for a bit right, it's not about the addiction to progression it is the progression in the conviction (ooh I like that) in keeping the body at this position for this duration of time you can almost guarantee the body will see this as it's new norm and you will be able to push on again after this period of reset in order to reach further goals along the journey you are on.

What happens when you do drop off? This is speaking from experience here and I want to dive into the reality of my mindset when I fell off the biggest journey I had ever been on at the start of dropping fat.

I was a lot younger but it messed with my head at unexplainable levels and lead to the start of a full on eating disorder. It was around 10 years ago now which I dropped nearly 100lbs and got onto the bodybuilding stage for the first time, I had dropped weight and then I had the final 42lb to lose in order to get stage ready, I gave myself 3 months in order to do this which was doable if you like crash dieting.

My exercise routine at this moment in time was 60-90 minutes cardio every morning during the week and 45 minutes every evening whilst weight training 5 times per week without fail, every single item of food was weighed out to the gram and the final 4-5 weeks I had literally no carbohydrates (you know, those sexy things which give you the stuff we love – energy). In fact it was at this point I was working in a gym and I remember going up the stairs I would get a head rush, even getting out of a chair too quickly it would happen and I would have to stand for about 10 seconds to get my bearings before moving on. One shift in particular I was working with a colleague who was the duty manager at the time so the gym was her responsibility, it also happens she was about 7 months pregnant, I remember going up the stairs after the gym had shut ready to do the cleaning, then I remember getting woken up, I had actually fallen asleep at the top of the stairs and made the lady who was heavily pregnant put all the weights away and clean everything, yeah, I felt like a dick.
I competed in my first bodybuilding show in August that year which I managed to proudly win a plastic trophy for coming in second place, that was cool but what wasn't cool was qualifying for the British finals, it meant another 8 weeks of dieting and was the turning point for me starting on my eating disorder.

I had over dieted, I remember my squat actually being a struggle at 60kg and falling over (for reference this morning I squatted 200kg for 3 reps around 80% effort) I was dropping weight but my body fat was seemingly increasing at the same time and the last straw was when I actually knew my mind was going due to the over dieting situation I had put myself in, I woke up about 4am one morning and drove to my dad's grave actually asking him for permission to stop this dieting and quit the road to the finals. Funny thing was I asked permission but nobody in the world had forced me to do it, it was all my own doing.

After this time – it was around the end of September when I finally called it quits on competing again that year – I had a bit of a fall off the wagon due to the large amount of restriction I had put myself through, binged for around a week and then got back onto a plan, loosely may I add. By Christmas I had put on nearly all of the weight I had lost, in fact, I had lost muscle so I had actually got back to a worst condition than I started back before the competition diet.

Add to this, I had just competed in the juniors that year and right then I couldn't get my dick to play ball no matter what I tried doing, I was depressed and hated even taking my top off in front of the mirror let alone with anyone else present. It took a long while to get my metabolism back on the ball from that point, around 6-8 months to put a number on it and because of this screw up I thought I was creating balance which definitely wasn't the case.

After realising how bad I rebounded and started the yo-yo process I never wanted to get into that position again, I dieted down over a longer period of time but it was still not healthy, not balanced, not sustainable to someone who has a life. I got shredded at the end of that year and kind of stayed like that for the next 6-7 years missing more social events than I can count on my fingers, cutting weddings short due to not being able to take my Tupperware, losing contact with friends and even nearly losing a job because of it. You know what I laugh at now but at the time it was a dumb thing to do? I took a girl on a first date to the cinema (yeah, how creative of me I know!) but I also took a Tupperware of broccoli and chicken all boiled up, it stunk, we didn't have a second date…

This is where the 'refine' phase is essential, well, the whole three phases, if I had used my own methods (which I did develop after this with these examples being some of the big reasons why they were developed) I wouldn't have had to fall off, I would have kept in the shape I was close to, I say close to purely because being in show condition year round isn't healthy in my opinion, I mean, is it really nice to have to have an extra cushion on your car seat because you have no fat on your arse and back that it actually hurts?!

This is why we need a 'refine' phase, we stop the yo-yoing and make sure that your results are consistent and guaranteed.

So now you know the reasons for each phase it is a case of just going all in making sure you Align, Design and Refine.

Align yourself to dive into your goals, why you want them, what happens when you get them, what happens if you don't get them.
Design your ideal life through your body, your health and your fitness, your SELF.

Refine the reality, don't fall into that crevasse, cycle your success and make sure it's a continuum of the journey you want to be on.

14. What Is It Really Like To Lose 100lbs?

"If we are not ashamed to think it, we should not be ashamed to say it." - Marcus Tullius Cicero

You have my guidelines, now let me tell you a little about my personal journey when I lost around 100lbs, what it really feels like, I think it will be a little bit of an eye opener.

Then I will leave you to decide what you will do with the information in this book, whether you action it or decide to just throw it back on your shelf, hard drive, kindle, whatever method you've read it by.

If you want to contact me you've been given my email multiple times, if you want to implement the actions but just need a little help, I am here for you ollie@revitalizationblueprint.com.

So what does losing 100lb actually feel like?

Is it as good as it sounds?

Let me go back to the beginning and describe my lifestyle, where I was and how I felt once I actually realised I had a problem.

Back when I was 15 my father passed away suddenly, he had a migraine the Wednesday and the Saturday he died from a stroke, it was a hard time for the whole family but it impacted me more than I knew it.

I was already a shy kid and when I went back for my final year at school things were different, there was a grown sense within me but I was getting bullied a lot for being who I was, the shy guy who loved hip hop and now my father had passed away, I am not sure the people in school were aware but it actually hit me very hard when they took digs and I heard someone say 'that's the geeky boy who's dad died' I had a name around the school it seemed, that hurt.

I didn't realize it at the time but I slowly turned to food as my emotional release, I was eating a lot, hiding wrappers in the trash and even just skipping lessons sometimes, going to the local store and filling up on sausage rolls and pastries, it was my safe place, all while listening to hip hop and going home to play video games for hours on end.

By the time I was around 19 years old I was morbidly obese, I was finding it hard to be confident with women and even though I had a couple of girlfriends before, it was hard, I would be so ashamed of letting them see me naked I would even have sex with the lights off and top on, I would even keep my top on in bed during the summer months when it was ridiculously hot outside.

Things had to change.

I remember walking to music college and getting out of breath, not a harsh walk, around 20 minutes from the car park, flat, no reason to be tired but I got there and it really hit me how much I had been hiding behind the food rather than facing up to the bereavement of losing a parent at a young age had put on me.

I started counselling.

It wasn't until a few session down the line and I was around 21 that my best friend at the time was into training asked if I wanted to go to the gym. When I say gym I mean local country club which was stuck in the 1980s and literally a small place to train, I went.

When I walking into the building I remember seeing what I thought were massive guys over at the free weight section (which went up to around 75lbs tops), people who 'knew what they were doing' in the smith machine and using the machines. I let Ash go do his thing and went on a treadmill, it all started then.

After a few sessions I asked for a program and still to this day, my first trainer is a friend of mine and coincidently he now comes to me for advice and he actually had to force me to accept money the last time as I feel he was vital for me to begin on this journey, Millsy, I will be forever greatful for the kick.

I sorted my nutrition, I thought, invested in some Slim Fast along with ready meals (you know the ones which everyone says give you bitch tits…they couldn't get any worse, what the heck!)

As things progressed I think I purchased a protein shake and god forbid

SOME CREATINE

But after a while things were moving nicely and I dropped a hell of a lot before jumping on a bodybuilding stage 10th August 2008.

OK I missed a lot out here but the point has only just begun.

Losing the weight was only the start of it, I was shredded.

I was at the goal I had always wanted to be, abs and I thought I loved it.

That was until a social event came and I had to eat off of my plan things were noticeably harder right now and psychologically my mind was fucked. I would find myself staring at the menu for days beforehand like a child watching Baywatch for the first time and wondering why the producers put Pamela Anderson in slow motion, or The Hoff, whatever imagery you want there take your pick. I would change my mind so much and still never decide until the time actually came to order as I was torn between having the nachos which have actually been proven that they are the food of gods or settling for the 8oz rump with a side of vegetables which have been proven it is errr well, just, steak really.

Then there was the fear creeping in my mind –

If I have the nachos will I just go back to where I started, the fat guy with more spare tires than a Nascar pit garage?

That was a horrible thought, the guilt, the fear, the emotions were beyond what I would even wish on my worst enemy. What if I had them and then I couldn't fit into my clothes, had to go back to a 42inch waist for my work wear?

What, what if I lost my partner because of eating nachos?

You may find it funny to believe but these were actual thoughts, thoughts that happened regularly when meals off the plan became a thing.

I remember one time I took a girl out on a date, first time trying to impress her I wouldn't even have a diet coke (they didn't have zero back then), I took my chicken and broccoli meal into the movie theatre and proceeded to munch away stinking the whole place out, she looked at me with disgust, we didn't have a second date.

Another relationship I started but wouldn't go out and drink, a nice lady who I really liked but after about 6 weeks things weren't great and she couldn't handle the fact of how restrained I was, these things all led to binging out because of the strict diet I was trying to follow.

Every once in around 3-4 weeks I would let loose and really go for it, my mum and step dad would moan as I would clear out most of the cupboard from cookies to ice cream and everything else I could literally get my hands on. The next 4-5 days I would add in extra cardio as all I could see in the mirror was that fat kid getting bullied, I would starve myself, oh, sorry…FAST for a 24 hour period to reset everything whilst taking a laxative to make sure I was shitting as much out as possible.

This is the way it went on for a few years, I had to get professional help in the end about the control I had around my relationship with food.

This is what my mind became because of one reason when I lost all that weight, I didn't have a mentor, I didn't have a coach or anyone to tell me the really simple way and what would happen when and if I done something.

It was nasty, I hated every second but made out like I was it was a happy ever after Monica and Chandler story starting out like you've never expect it to happen then BOOM – I'll be there for you, it was at the forefront of my mind, my life, my existence (wait, did Monica and Chandler stay together?).

It took time to get over this and I find it is something I relate to with so many people, so many clients come to me because they know how I 'get it' they may have the weight to lose but know how I made the mistake in the past, they may have lost the weight and want to get to that next level and find the knowledge I have had from going through this stuff to be priceless.

What is it you need to do in order to get through your weight loss journey stronger and in the place you want to be?

What is it you need in ore to really upgrade yourself?

What is it you need to accomplish to be able to walk through your One Day Body Upgrade?

Who do you need to become?

Ask yourself these questions.

When you need to talk further about it then please don't hesitate about getting in touch, I am here
www.revitalizationblueprint.com/letstalk

About The Author

In the beginning Ollie lost his father, a traumatic time led to extensive emotional eating making the weight shoot up to 250lbs and more, it was then where Ollie was working in a corporate job and when being a 'successful guy' was mentioned this was the furthest anyone could possibly be – low confidence, high body fat, no sales skills, no morale.

When having sex and not wanting to take his top off it finally hit him, he needed to do something about it and got a membership at the gym, invested in his own personal trainer (who coincidently Ollie now mentors himself), this was the start of a massive chapter.

Ollie left the corporate world to add fitness as his job and swiftly dropped nearly 100lbs in 12 months to step onto a bodybuilding stage, it was here that learning about nutrition became vital, everything that could be taken on board was taken on board, every hack, every secret, every method was tried to find out what was best to drop weight and put on muscle. This had a dramatic impact on Ollie's life after 4 years doing this full time he was offered a position back in his previous job and how times had changed.

Within 6 months of accepting the job Ollie was the top sales guy in the company, this self-confident, powerful and driven individual could not be recognised when compared to his former self, fitness had literally laid the path to be the successful guy everyone was talking about within the company, this was great and it led to Ollie becoming a manager leading over 30 people at any one time.

This wasn't enough, Ollie had found his passion with his time in the fitness industry and this made him hungry, he was Revitalized and had unfinished business after helping multiple people online he decided to take the leap and go back full time with this new attitude.

Ollie has now worked with people all over the world and having been brought up in a family full of endurance athletes actually became 'that guy' for nutrition in endurance working with Olympic athletes, world champion triathletes and even Tour De France riders whilst training personally in both strength and endurance himself knowing the importance of constant self development in all areas.

It was when looking back on the story of his father passing away before his time that he realized his calling. You see, his father was only trying to provide for his family, working his ass off and financial he was definitely providing but what was missing was the focus on his health, at 47 years old Trevor Matthews passed away suffering a stroke which, with a little more focus on both stress management and health from the inside out could potentially have been prevented.

Not focusing on health stopped Ollie's father from seeing massive events in his life – both Ollie and his sister's wedding days, granddaughter being born, graduations and even just literally going for a drive on a Sunday afternoon to watch the game.

The Revitalization Blueprint is who Ollie is, it is who Ollie's clients are and the development of The Revitalized Blueprint: Intensive has literally changed the game, there is nothing else more important than yourself, this is why, as mentioned at the start, Ollie is the guy who practices what he preaches.

Thank You's

This isn't a thank you just for releasing a book, this is much more, this is a thank you for allowing me to be where I am today, if you feel you deserve to be on this list but I have missed you, sorry and thank you anyway too.

Dad – The guy who I look up to every single day and wish that I could have just one more second with you.

Mum – Thanks for being you, I may lose patience but you're always there.

Gav – My step dad, you didn't have to step in the way you did but thank you, it takes a lot to show the love you have to both myself and Ellie.

Ellie – Big sis, just keep running, just…keep…running

Laura – We may have been through some struggles but thank you for being there when I need.

Dexter & Snowy – It's not a thank you without thanking your dogs is it?

DJ – My best mate since go knows how young we were, cheers for being there.

Nick Wilson – You were my first paying PT client when I wasn't allowed to charge at Wensum, now you're one of my best friends.

Wayne Crowe – It's great to know another likeminded individual locally, we are never alone, work Christmas party is happening this year.

Mark Claxton – I wouldn't have got on stage back in 2008 if it wasn't for your help, you moody fuck.

Rob Cox – Beast mode activated! Those Brum trips were legendary.

Lee Shorten – Thanks for being there man.

Mark Bone & Shaun Tester – Thank you both for managing Bodyrush and now Phoenix Gym

Lindsey Anderson – The support you gave me to leave my role at Aviva was amazing, one of the best bosses I have ever had.

Iain Mills – My first trainer, it's great to be able to give back to you now.

Barbs Murray – From my first personal training case study it's been an amazing journey, even if we don't see each other as much as we say we should.

Matt Fever – Helping me through my level 3 personal training course.

Lisa Atthowe – Yes, I am going to thank and ex, it's my book and Lisa if you read this thanks for supporting me through my first big weight loss and competition, I was pretty fucked most of that prep!

Dan Meredith – My bearded brother from another mother, still proud to this day to have been one of your first online coaching clients, anytime you need me just call.

Ron Reich – You're getting a special mention as my A-Player client, friend and also a mentor, thanks.

John Romaniello – After looking up to you for so long it's great to be mentored by you.

John Cusick – I would 100% never have believed I could do an MSc without your crazy chats, you are one of the most genuine and caring people I know.

Shari Teigman – Crazy New Jersey lady! Love you and thanks for being so fucking epic!

Mark Whitehand – LORD! You and your stories have got me

into places I found it hard to get out of!

Joe Gregory – This wouldn't have been created without you, thanks.

Billy Hopkins – You're an amazing guy, always remember that and not matter what I will always have time for you my scouse brother!

Alex Viada – One of the best things I asked was to be coached by you and ended up becoming a Complete Human Performance coach! Thanks for being a great mentor.

Alex Harris – You believed when I said there was 12 weeks to a bodybuilding show, and even travelled 100s of miles to get there, you will always be a great friend bro.

Steve Gibbons – Amazing to see someone doing so well in Norwich, some great chats already between us.

John Chapman & Leon Bustin – You guys are beyond inspirational and still thank you for taking me to Cliff & Marta's seminar.

Stephen Aish – Socrates, I am here, now.

Cliff & Marta Wilde – Just thank you DOODES! AWESOME!

Adil Amarsi – You're one of the good guys, glad to call you a friend.

Hollis Carter – Thanks for believing in me to be the trainer at Baby Bathwater

Emil Goliath – Epic to know someone doing similar things which we know is just going to help millions of people.

Steven Eugene Kuhn – Brother, it's not been long but the love is so strong.

Sam Shaw – You were the partner in rhyme allowing me to start to build my confidence up, maybe we shouldn't have had to many UK Pizza though!

Ahmed Abdelmutti – We have some stories and thanks for being my boy back in the day.

Thando Murwira – Whats Good? Whats Realllllly Good? What's really really really really good? You know!

Ashley Scott – You helped me get to Wensum that first time.

Robby Copsey – One of my best mates in school, those English lessons writing rhymes are paying off!

Lee Guyton – RZ for life.

To some amazing clients I have been able to work with:

Doberman Dan

Ron Reich - yeah second mention!

Ryan McKenzie - Some of our WhatsApp conversations are pretty 'different' coaching topics!

Adam Lundquist – Thanks for being a friend and great client too.

Rick Barker – I have learned so much just from being able to coach you and call you a friend.

Hannah Pennington – One of the first people to ever sign up to my online coaching and proud to have you as my official photographer and videographer.

Adam Killam
John Pagulayan
Phill Sardi
Phil Powis
Eddys Velasguez
Taylor Draper
Dean Watts

Jack Mason
Kristin Moura
Tracey Aldous
Tony Peck

And many more

As I said, apologies if I missed anyone.
Thank you all.

Printed in Great Britain
by Amazon